Role of Sexual Abuse in the Etiology of Borderline Personality Disorder

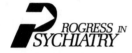

PROGRESS IN PSYCHIATRY

David Spiegel, M.D.
Series Editor

Role of Sexual Abuse in the Etiology of Borderline Personality Disorder

Edited by
Mary C. Zanarini, Ed.D.

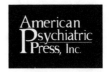

Washington, DC
London, England

Copyright © 1997 American Psychiatric Press, Inc.

ALL RIGHTS RESERVED

Manufactured in the United States of America on acid-free paper

First Edition   00   99   98   97   4   3   2   1

American Psychiatric Press, Inc.
1400 K Street, N.W., Washington, DC   20005

Library of Congress Cataloging-in-Publication Data

Role of sexual abuse in etiology of borderline personality disorder /
   edited by Mary C. Zanarini.—1st ed.
         p.   cm.—(Progress in Psychiatry ; #49)
      Includes bibliographical references and index.
      ISBN 0-88048-496-9 (alk. paper)
      1. Borderline personality disorder—Etiology.   2. Adult child
   sexual abuse victims—Mental health.   I. Zanarini, Mary C., 1946-
   II. Series.
      [DNLM: 1. Borderline Personality Disorder—etiology. 2. Child
   Abuse, Sexual—psychology. W1 PR6781L no.49 1997 / WM 190 R745
   1997]
   RC569.5.B67R65 1997
   616.85'852071—dc20
   DNLM/DLC
   for Library of Congress   95-26270
                                                                    CIP

British Library Cataloguing in Publication Data
A CIP record is available from the British Library.

Contents

Introduction to the Progress in Psychiatry Series   vii

Contributors   ix

1   Evolving Perspectives on the Etiology of
Borderline Personality Disorder   1
Mary C. Zanarini, Ed.D.

2   Parameters of Childhood Sexual Abuse in
Female Patients   15
Joel Paris, M.D., and Hallie Zweig-Frank, Ph.D.

3   Childhood Factors Associated With the
Development of Borderline Personality Disorder   29
*Mary C. Zanarini, Ed.D., Elyse D. Dubo, M.D.,
F.R.C.P.(C.), Ruth E. Lewis, Ph.D., and
Amy A. Williams, B.S.*

4   Etiological Factors in a Sample of Convicted
Women Felons in North Carolina   45
*B. Kathleen Jordan, Ph.D., William E. Schlenger,
Ph.D., Juesta M. Caddell, Ph.D., and John A.
Fairbank, Ph.D.*

5   Relationship of Childhood Abuse and
Maternal Attachment to the Development of
Borderline Personality Disorder   71
*Judith P. Salzman, Ed.D., Carl Salzman, M.D.,
and Abbie N. Wolfson, M.A.*

6   Relationship of Childhood Sexual Abuse to
Dissociation and Self-Mutilation in
Female Patients   93
Hallie Zweig-Frank, Ph.D., and Joel Paris, M.D.

7 Relationship Between Lifetime
   Self-Destructiveness and Pathological
   Childhood Experiences   107
   Elyse D. Dubo, M.D., F.R.C.P.(C.), Mary C.
   Zanarini, Ed.D., Ruth E. Lewis, Ph.D., and
   Amy A. Williams, B.S.

8 Severity of Childhood Sexual Abuse, Borderline
   Symptoms, and Familial Environment   131
   Kenneth R. Silk, M.D., Joel T. Nigg, Ph.D.,
   Drew Westen, Ph.D., and Naomi E. Lohr, Ph.D.

9 Neurological Vulnerability and Trauma in
   Borderline Personality Disorder   165
   Catherine Rising Kimble, M.D., Godehard
   Oepen, M.D., Elizabeth Weinberg, M.D.,
   Amy A. Williams, B.S., and Mary C.
   Zanarini, Ed.D.

10 A History of Childhood Sexual Abuse and
   the Course of Borderline Personality Disorder   181
   M. Janice E. Mitton, R.N., B.A., M.H.Sc.,
   Paul S. Links, M.D., F.R.C.P.(C.), M.Sc., and
   Gerald Durocher, B.A., M.A.

11 Biosocial Perspective on the Relationship of
   Childhood Sexual Abuse, Suicidal Behavior,
   and Borderline Personality Disorder   203
   Amy W. Wagner, Ph.D., and Marsha M.
   Linehan, Ph.D.

12 Effects of a History of Childhood Abuse on
   Treatment of Borderline Patients   225
   John G. Gunderson, M.D.

   Index   237

Introduction to the
Progress in Psychiatry Series

The Progress in Psychiatry Series is designed to capture in print the excitement that comes from assembling a diverse group of experts from various locations to examine in detail the newest information about a developing aspect of psychiatry. This series emerged as a collaboration between the American Psychiatric Association's (APA) Scientific Program Committee and the American Psychiatric Press, Inc. Great interest is generated by a number of the symposia presented each year at the APA annual meeting, and we realized that much of the information presented there, carefully assembled by people who are deeply immersed in a given area, would unfortunately not appear together in print. The symposia sessions at the annual meetings provide an unusual opportunity for experts who otherwise might not meet on the same platform to share their diverse viewpoints for a period of 3 hours. Some new themes are repeatedly reinforced and gain credence, whereas in other instances disagreements emerge, enabling the audience and now the reader to reach informed decisions about new directions in the field. The Progress in Psychiatry Series allows us to publish and capture some of the best of the symposia and thus provide an in-depth treatment of specific areas that might not otherwise be presented in broader review formats.

Psychiatry is, by nature, an interface discipline, combining the study of mind and brain, of individual and social environments, of the humane and the scientific. Therefore, progress in the field is rarely linear—it often comes from unexpected sources. Furthermore, new developments emerge from an array of viewpoints that do not necessarily provide immediate agreement but rather expert examination of the issues. We intend to present innovative ideas and data that will enable you, the reader, to participate in this process.

We believe the Progress in Psychiatry Series will provide you with an opportunity to review timely, new information in specific fields of interest as they are developing. We hope you find that the excitement of the presentations is captured in the written word and that this book proves to be informative and enjoyable reading.

David Spiegel, M.D.
Series Editor
Progress in Psychiatry Series

Contributors

Juesta M. Caddell, Ph.D.
Clinical Research Psychologist, Research Triangle Institute, Research Triangle Park, North Carolina

Elyse D. Dubo, M.D., F.R.C.P.(C.)
Assistant Professor of Psychiatry, University of Toronto, Sunnybrook Health Sciences Centre, Toronto, Ontario, Canada

Gerald Durocher, B.A., M.A.
Psychometrist, Department of Research, Hamilton Psychiatric Hospital, Hamilton, Ontario, Canada

John A. Fairbank, Ph.D.
Senior Clinical Research Psychologist, Research Triangle Institute, Research Triangle Park, North Carolina

John G. Gunderson, M.D.
Director, Psychosocial Research and Training Program, McLean Hospital, Belmont, Massachusetts; Professor of Psychiatry, Harvard Medical School, Boston, Massachusetts

B. Kathleen Jordan, Ph.D.
Senior Research Sociologist, Research Triangle Institute, Research Triangle Park, North Carolina

Catherine Rising Kimble, M.D.
Assistant Attending Psychiatrist, McLean Hospital, Belmont, Massachusetts; Clinical Instructor in Psychiatry, Harvard Medical School, Boston, Massachusetts

Ruth E. Lewis, Ph.D.
Clinical and Research Fellow in Psychology, McLean Hospital, Belmont, Massachusetts; Harvard Medical School, Boston, Massachusetts

Marsha M. Linehan, Ph.D.
Professor, Department of Psychology, University of
Washington, Seattle, Washington

Paul S. Links, M.D., F.R.C.P.(C.), M.Sc.
Professor of Psychiatry, University of Toronto, Wellesley
Hospital, Toronto, Ontario, Canada

Naomi E. Lohr, Ph.D.
Assistant Professor of Psychiatry and Psychology,
Departments of Psychiatry and Psychology, University of
Michigan, Ann Arbor, Michigan

M. Janice E. Mitton, R.N., B.A., M.H.Sc.
Clinical Lecturer, Department of Psychiatry, McMaster
University, Hamilton, Ontario, Canada

Joel T. Nigg, Ph.D.
Assistant Professor, Department of Psychology,
Michigan State University,
East Lansing, Michigan

Godehard Oepen, M.D.
Associate Professor of Psychiatry, Boston University School
of Medicine, Boston, Massachusetts

Joel Paris, M.D.
Professor, Department of Psychiatry, McGill University;
Research Associate, Institute of Community and Family
Psychiatry, Sir Mortimer B. Davis–Jewish General Hospital,
Montreal, Quebec, Canada

Carl Salzman, M.D.
Professor of Psychiatry, Massachusetts Mental
Health Center, Harvard Medical School, Boston,
Massachusetts

Judith P. Salzman, Ed.D.
Research Associate, Massachusetts Mental Health Center,
Harvard Medical School, Boston, Massachusetts

William E. Schlenger, Ph.D.
Senior Research Psychologist and Director, Mental and Behavioral Health Research Program, Research Triangle Institute, Research Triangle Park, North Carolina

Kenneth R. Silk, M.D.
Associate Professor and Associate Chair for Clinical and Administrative Affairs, Department of Psychiatry, University of Michigan Medical Center, Ann Arbor, Michigan

Amy W. Wagner, Ph.D.
Women's Health Sciences Division, National Center for PTSD, Boston VA Medical Center, Boston, Massachusetts

Elizabeth Weinberg, M.D.
Assistant Professor of Psychiatry, Baylor College of Medicine, Houston, Texas

Drew Westen, Ph.D.
Chief Psychologist, Cambridge Hospital, Cambridge, Massachusetts; Associate Professor of Psychology, Harvard Medical School, Boston, Massachusetts

Amy A. Williams, B.S.
Department of Psychology, New York University, New York, New York; Senior Clinical Coordinator, McLean Study of Adult Development, McLean Hospital, Belmont, Massachusetts

Abbie N. Wolfson, M.A.
Department of Psychology, Boston University, Boston, Massachusetts

Mary C. Zanarini, Ed.D.
Director, McLean Study of Adult Development and Laboratory for the Study of Adult Development, McLean Hospital, Belmont, Massachusetts; Assistant Professor of Psychology, Harvard Medical School, Boston, Massachusetts

Hallie Zweig-Frank, Ph.D.
Associate Professor of Psychology, Concordia University; Research Associate, Institute of Community and Family Psychiatry, Sir Mortimer B. Davis–Jewish General Hospital, Montreal, Quebec, Canada

Chapter 1

Evolving Perspectives on the Etiology of Borderline Personality Disorder

Mary C. Zanarini, Ed.D.

The place of borderline personality disorder (BPD) in psychiatric nosology has long been a point of contention. Stern (1938) was the first author to use the term *borderline* to describe a specific pathological condition—a condition that he thought had both neurotic and psychotic features. Since that time there have been six main conceptualizations of this term. The first of these is based on the work of Kernberg (1975). In this view, the term *borderline* is used to describe most serious forms of character pathology. The second conceptualization reflects the work of Gunderson (1984). In this view, the term *borderline* describes a specific form of personality disorder that can be distinguished from a substantial number of other Axis II disorders, particularly those in the "odd" and "anxious" clusters of DSM-III and DSM-III-R (American Psychiatric Association 1980, 1987). The third conceptualization, which flourished in the 1960s and 1970s, focused on the propensity of borderline patients to have transient psychotic or psychotic-like experiences. In this view, borderline personality was thought of as being a schizophrenia spectrum disorder (Wender 1977). The fourth conceptualization, which organized much of clinical care and empirical research in the 1980s, focused on the chronic dysphoria and affective lability

Supported in part by National Institute of Mental Health grant MH47588.

1

of borderline patients. In this view, borderline personality was thought of as being an affective spectrum disorder (Akiskal 1981; Stone 1980).

Both the fifth and sixth theories of borderline psychopathology have arisen during the 1990s.

Zanarini (1993) proposed the fifth theory—that borderline personality disorder is best conceptualized as an impulse spectrum disorder (i.e., a disorder related to substance use disorders, antisocial personality disorder, and perhaps eating disorders). In this view, BPD is not seen as an attenuated or atypical form of one of these impulse spectrum disorders. Rather, it is suggested that BPD is a specific form of personality disorder that may share a propensity to action with other disorders of impulse control.

During the late 1980s and early 1990s, a number of studies found elevated rates of BPD among survivors of childhood sexual abuse (Briere and Zaidi 1989; Herman 1986). These reports served as the empirical basis for the sixth theory—that BPD is a trauma spectrum disorder, related to posttraumatic stress disorder and dissociative disorders, including multiple personality disorder (Herman and van der Kolk 1987).

Despite these differing views of BPD, the diagnosis is now a well-established part of official nomenclature. It is also the best-validated Axis II disorder with the exception of antisocial personality disorder (Pope et al. 1983; Zanarini et al. 1990).

PSYCHODYNAMIC THEORIES OF THE PATHOGENESIS OF BPD

Although the validity of BPD is now generally accepted, the etiology of the disorder is still in the process of being uncovered. The first attempt to explain the development of BPD came from the psychoanalytic community, and over the years, three major psychodynamic theories of the pathogenesis of the disorder have been proposed.

In the first of these theories, Kernberg (1975) suggested that excessive early aggression leads the young child to split his positive and negative images of himself and his mother. This excess aggression may have been inborn, or it may have been caused by real frustrations. In either case, the preborderline child is unable to merge her positive and negative images and attendant affects to achieve a more realistic and ambivalent view of herself and others.

In the second of these theories, Adler and Buie (1979) suggested that failures in early mothering led to a child's failure to develop stable object constancy. Because the preborderline child's mothering was inconsistent and often insensitive and nonempathic, the child fails to develop a consistent view of himself or others that he can use in times of stress to comfort and sustain himself.

In the third of these theories, Masterson (1972) suggested that fear of abandonment is the central factor in borderline psychopathology. He believed that the mother of the future borderline patient interfered with her child's natural autonomous strivings by withdrawing emotionally when the child acted in an independent manner during the phase of development that Mahler (1971) has termed *separation-individuation*. Later experiences that require independent behavior lead to a recrudescence of the dysphoria and the abandonment panic that the borderline patient felt as a child when faced with a seemingly insoluble dilemma (either continue to behave dependently or lose needed emotional support).

FIRST-GENERATION STUDIES OF THE PATHOGENESIS OF BPD

The first generation of studies of the environmental factors that might be of etiological significance for BPD focused on issues raised in the psychodynamic theories reviewed above. Two topics were studied with particular care: parental separation or loss and disturbed parental involvement.

Parental Separation or Loss

In a small study of a part of the sample in Grinker et al. (1968), Walsh (1977) found that a majority of families of borderline patients (57%) had histories of parental loss through divorce or death—a significantly higher percentage than was found in a group of matched control subjects with schizophrenia. In addition, half the borderline patients had experienced a serious chronic parental illness that often required extensive hospitalization. Only 21% of the patients with BPD came from families that had not experienced the loss of a parent through death, divorce, or serious illness. In another small study, Bradley (1979) found that the majority (64%) of children or adolescents with BPD had had prolonged separations in the first 5 years of life and that they were significantly more likely to have had such separations than were control subjects with either psychosis or a personality disorder. Soloff and Millward (1983) compared separation experiences in the backgrounds of 45 patients with BPD with those of comparison groups with depression and schizophrenia. They found that the patients with BPD were significantly more likely to come from single-parent families than were those in either control group. They also found that patients with BPD had a significantly higher incidence of loss of their fathers by divorce or death (47%). Akiskal et al. (1985) found that 37% of borderline patients had experienced a developmentally important loss—a percentage significantly higher than that of control subjects with affective disorders and significantly lower than that of control subjects with personality disorders.

Disturbed Parental Involvement

The original study characterizing the families of borderline patients (Grinker et al. 1968) found that a minority (12.8%, or 6/47 families) were characterized by relationships in which the parents were overinvolved and overprotective. Another 19.2% (9/47 families) were characterized by a pervasive denial of problems, which was evidenced by the absence of marital discord and the lack of strong parental affect of either a positive or negative nature. However, the most common pattern observed in these families (about a third, or 19/47 families) was a high degree of discord between the mother and her children and between the two parents.

Subsequently, Walsh (1977) found that a greater percentage (57%, or 8/14) of patients with BPD felt that they had been overinvolved with one parent, with whom they had had a special relationship. This relationship was judged as supportive of the parent's need to be needed but destructive to the patient's need to have a life of her own. Walsh also found that most (86%, or 12/14) of the borderline patients characterized their relationship with one or both parents as remote or lacking in feelings of attachment. In addition, she found that 64% (9/14) of her borderline cohort reported strongly negative, highly conflictual relationships with their parents, characterized by parental hostility, devaluation, or frank abuse.

Gunderson and colleagues (1980) studied three groups of patients who had had intact families: those with borderline personality, paranoid schizophrenia, and neurosis/other Axis II disorders. The parents of borderline patients were less likely than those of patients with neurosis but more likely than those of patients with schizophrenia to invest in their children at the expense of their marriage. More generally, results for the borderline patients failed to show a high level of overinvolved families but rather found that the parents had been involved with each other to the exclusion of their children.

Frank and Paris (1981) compared the accounts of parental attitudes of three samples: those with BPD, those with neuroses/other personality disorders, and psychiatrically healthy control subjects. All three groups reported disturbed attitudes in their mothers. The borderline group remembered their fathers as being significantly less interested in and less approving of them in general than did the other two groups. Their fathers, more specifically, were reported to be less interested in and less approving of dependent behaviors than fathers of control subjects with neuroses/other personality disorders. In a subsequent small study, Frank and Hoffman (1986) found that females with BPD remembered both their mothers and their fathers as being significantly less nurturant and less affectionate than did neurotic control subjects. In a third study by this group, Paris and Frank (1989) found that borderline women perceived their parents as being significantly less caring than did woman control subjects.

Soloff and Millward (1983) found that inpatients with BPD, as well as control subjects with depression and schizophrenia, saw their mothers as being overinvolved with them. The patients with BPD were, however, significantly more likely to see their fathers as being underinvolved than were patients from either control group. Soloff and Millward also reported that the borderline patients saw their relationships with their mothers and fathers as being significantly more negative and conflictual than did the two control groups.

Goldberg and colleagues (1985) retrospectively assessed with a self-report questionnaire the parental attitudes of 24 patients with BPD, 22 general psychiatric control subjects, and 10 psychiatrically healthy control subjects. They found that patients with BPD remembered both their parents as being significantly less caring than did those in either control group. They also found that patients with BPD remembered their parents as being significantly more overprotective than did the psychiatrically healthy control subjects.

Four conclusions emerged from these studies: 1) prolonged childhood separations are both common and discriminating for patients with borderline personality; 2) patients with BPD usually see their relationships with their mothers as highly conflictual, distant, or uninvolved; 3) the father's failure to be present and involved is an even more discriminating aspect of these families than are the mother's problems; and 4) disturbed relationships with both parents may be more specific for BPD and more pathogenic than a disturbed relationship with either one alone.

SECOND-GENERATION STUDIES OF
THE PATHOGENESIS OF BPD

The second generation of studies of the environmental factors that may be pathogenic for BPD built upon the methodological limitations of the studies reviewed in the previous section. Most of the second-generation studies reviewed below (Table 1–1) have incorporated the following three methodological advances: 1) diagnoses were determined through semistructured interviews, 2) childhood experiences were assessed through semistructured interviews, and 3) diagnostic information and childhood information were obtained, each blind to information

Table 1–1. Prevalence of childhood physical and sexual abuse in criteria-defined borderline patients

Study	BPD N	Control subjects	Treatment status	Gender	Physical abuse	Caretaker sexual abuse	Overall sexual abuse
Links et al. 1988	88	42 BPD trait	Inpatients	Mixed	29[a]	26[a]	—
Herman et al. 1989	21	34 mixed	Outpatients/symptomatic volunteers	Mixed	71	—	67[a]
Zanarini et al. 1989	50	55 Axis II	Outpatients	Mixed	46	26[a]	—
Ogata et al. 1990	24	18 depressed	Inpatients	Mixed	42	25	71[a]
Shearer et al. 1990	40	—	Inpatients	Female	25	28	40
Westen et al. 1990	27	23 mixed	Inpatients	Female	52	33	52[a]
Salzman et al. 1993	31	—	Symptomatic volunteers	Mixed	10	0	16

[a]Reported by a significantly higher percentage of borderline patients than control subjects.

pertaining to the other domain. Second-generation studies have also tended to focus more on childhood experiences of abuse than on childhood experiences of parental loss and disturbed parental involvement. Links et al. (1988) and Zanarini et al. (1989) published their results almost simultaneously. Links et al. compared the childhood experiences of 88 borderline inpatients with those of 42 inpatients with borderline traits. They found that borderline patients were significantly more likely than control subjects to report being sexually abused by a caretaker, being physically abused by a caretaker, and being separated from their primary caretaker for a period of 3 months or more. Zanarini et al. compared the childhood experiences of 50 borderline outpatients with those of 55 outpatient control subjects with DSM Axis II disorders. They found that a significantly higher percentage of borderline patients than Axis II control subjects reported being verbally abused and sexually abused by a caretaker before the age of 18. They also found that rates of physical abuse by caretakers and three forms of caretaker neglect (physical neglect, emotional withdrawal, and inconsistent treatment) did not significantly distinguish borderline patients from Axis II control subjects. In terms of early separations that lasted 1 month or more, about equal percentages of borderline patients and Axis II control subjects reported such a separation from a caretaker before the age of 6. However, when the control subjects were broken down into those who met DSM-III criteria for antisocial personality disorder (who were mostly men) and those who met DSM-III criteria for dysthymic disorder plus some other form of personality disorder (who were mostly women), a significantly higher percentage of borderline than antisocial patients reported at least one such early-childhood separation. A significantly higher percentage of borderline than antisocial patients also reported that a caretaker had withdrawn from them emotionally.

Herman et al. (1989) compared the childhood histories of physical and sexual abuse of 21 borderline outpatients/symptomatic volunteers with those of 34 mixed subjects, 11 with borderline traits and 23 with other Axis II disorders or bipolar II disorder. When the patients were compared ordinally (by summing across age periods), both physical and sexual abuse before the age of

19 were significantly more common among borderline patients than among control subjects. However, when patients were compared nominally (positive or negative history of each type of abuse), sexual abuse continued to significantly distinguish borderline patients from control subjects, but physical abuse no longer successfully distinguished the groups.

Ogata et al. (1990) compared the childhood experiences of 24 borderline inpatients with those of 18 depressed inpatients. They found that a significantly higher percentage of borderline patients than control subjects reported being sexually abused during childhood and/or adolescence. They also found that borderline patients reported a high rate of physical abuse and a low rate of physical neglect. However, neither type of pathological experience was significantly more common among borderline patients than among control subjects. In terms of the parameters of abuse, 21% (5) of the borderline patients reported being abused by their father, 4% (1) by their mother, 29% (7) by a sibling, 25% (6) by another relative, and 50% (12) by a nonrelative. Of those abused, 53% (9) reported being abused by multiple perpetrators, and 41% (7) reported penetration. The average age at onset of abuse was between 7 and 10 years (depending on the relationship to the abuser).

Westen et al. (1990) studied the childhood experiences of 50 female adolescent inpatients. They found that a significantly higher percentage of the 27 borderline subjects than of the 23 control subjects (mixed psychiatric disorders) reported a childhood history of sexual abuse and physical neglect. Physical abuse, although common, did not significantly distinguish the two groups. In terms of the parameters of abuse, 29.6% (8) of the borderline patients reported being sexually abused by their fathers, 7.4% (2) by their mothers, and 40.7% (11) by others. In terms of these other types of abusers, 25.9% (7) of the borderline patients reported being abused by neighbors and friends, 7.4% (2) by siblings, and 7.4% (2) by extended family members. Again, most of the sexual abuse started during the latency years.

Both Shearer et al. (1990) and Salzman et al. (1993) conducted uncontrolled studies of the childhood experiences of borderline patients. Shearer et al. studied 40 female inpatients, and Salzman et al. studied 31 symptomatic volunteers representing the mild end of the outpatient borderline continuum. Shearer et al. found that 40.0% (16) of the borderline cohort reported being sexually abused by a nonpeer before the age of 15, 27.5% (11) reported some type of incest, 17.5% (7) reported particularly severe sexual abuse, and 25% (10) reported being physically abused to the point of injury. Salzman et al. found that 16.1% (5) of their borderline patients reported being sexually abused during childhood and that 9.7% (3) reported a childhood history of physical abuse. No patients reported being sexually abused by a caretaker, and only 1 reported being sexually abused by a relative.

Three main findings have emerged from these studies. First, both physical and sexual abuse are relatively common in the childhood histories of criteria-defined borderline patients. Second, physical abuse is generally not reported significantly more often by borderline patients than by control subjects. Third, sexual abuse is consistently reported significantly more often by borderline patients than by control subjects with depression or personality disorders.

TOWARD A THIRD GENERATION OF
STUDIES OF THE PATHOGENESIS OF BPD

Many of the chapters in this book represent the start of a third generation of studies of the etiology of BPD. They share a number of conceptual and methodological features. Most important among these features are a tendency to assess a range of pathological childhood experiences rather than to focus solely on the prevalence of sexual abuse, a tendency to explore more explicitly the important parameters of sexual abuse, and a tendency to use multivariate analyses in determining significant findings.

In this book, Paris and Frank discuss their exploration of the parameters of sexual abuse in a well-defined group of borderline outpatients, which found that childhood sexual abuse had a low specificity for BPD and that only a subgroup of borderline patients reported severe abuse experiences. Zanarini and colleagues report that they assessed the prevalence of a wide range of pathological childhood experiences and found that sexual abuse seemed to be an important factor in the etiology of BPD but that other factors, particularly neglect by caretakers of both genders, also played an important role. Jordan and colleagues report that they explored the role of sexual abuse in a group of borderline women imprisoned for committing a felony, which found that a variety of environmental factors, including a childhood history of sexual abuse, are risk factors for BPD. Salzman et al. present data from two studies of borderline outpatients and suggest that the development of mild forms of BPD is more closely associated with disordered childhood attachment patterns than with a childhood history of physical and/or sexual abuse.

Frank and Paris describe their study of the relationship between a childhood history of physical and sexual abuse and an adult pattern of self-mutilation and dissociation, finding that both self-mutilation and dissociation are more strongly related to the diagnosis of BPD than to histories of physical or sexual abuse. Dubo and colleagues report that they examined the parameters of lifetime self-destructiveness for a group of borderline inpatients, finding that this trait is related to childhood experiences of both abuse and neglect. Silk and colleagues review a series of studies conducted by their group that pointed to a relationship between a childhood history of abuse and the severity of the expression of certain sectors of borderline psychopathology. Kimble et al. report on their assessment of the neurodevelopmental histories of a group of borderline women and Axis II control subjects, which found that neurodevelopmental vulnerability is a stronger predictor of a borderline diagnosis than is a childhood history of sexual abuse. Mitton and Links report that they compared the short-term outcomes of borderline patients who had and had not been sexually abused by a caretaker and found that the abused borderline patients had a modestly poorer outcome than did the nonabused borderline patients.

Wagner and Linehan describe the role of childhood sexual abuse in the pathogenesis of BPD from the vantage point of Linehan's Dialectical Behavior Therapy, suggesting that it is a prototypical, although not necessary, invalidating experience. Gunderson (1984) discusses the treatment of borderline patients with a childhood history of abuse and suggests, in a major departure from his previous work, that a practical case manager approach is more likely, at least initially, to be successful than is psychodynamically oriented psychotherapy.

CAUTIONARY NOTE

This book is being published at a time when childhood sexual abuse is being suggested by some as the main etiological factor in almost all disorders common in women (Bass and Davis 1988; Blume 1990). It is also being published at a time when a substantial backlash or correcting influence to this view is being felt. Although some observers are merely cautioning against a simplistic view of the development of psychopathology, others are beginning to question the veracity of some accounts of childhood sexual abuse, particularly those involving repressed or dissociated memories (Loftus 1993).

Taken together, the available empirical evidence suggests that for some borderline patients, childhood sexual abuse is not an issue; for others, it is an important factor in the development of their subjective pain and objective psychopathology; and for yet another group, it may well have been the defining environmental factor in the etiology of their distress and "dis-ease."

Future research will more carefully explicate the relationship between a history of childhood sexual abuse and the later development of BPD. Future research will also explore a series of models implicating a complex, multidimensional etiology for this disorder. In the meantime, we need to listen carefully to what our patients are telling us and not fail them by denying what they have to say or compelling them to tell us what we want to hear. Their pain and their future well-being are what is important, not our need to defend closely held theoretical positions.

REFERENCES

Adler G, Buie D: Aloneness and borderline psychopathology: the possible relevance of child developmental issues. Int J Psychoanal 60:83–96, 1979

Akiskal HS: Subaffective disorders: dysthymic, cyclothymic and bipolar II disorders in the "borderline" realm. Psychiatr Clin North Am 4:25–46, 1981

Akiskal HS, Chen SE, Davis GC, et al: Borderline: an adjective in search of a noun. J Clin Psychiatry 46:41–48, 1985

American Psychiatric Association: Diagnostic and Statistical Manual of Mental Disorders, 3rd Edition. Washington, DC, American Psychiatric Association, 1980

American Psychiatric Association: Diagnostic and Statistical Manual of Mental Disorders, 3rd Edition, Revised. Washington, DC, American Psychiatric Association, 1987

Bass E, Davis L: The Courage to Heal. New York, Harper & Row, 1988

Blume ES: Secret Survivors: Uncovering Incest and Its Aftereffects in Women. New York, Wiley, 1990

Bradley SJ: The relationship of early maternal separation to borderline personality in children and adolescents: a pilot study. Am J Psychiatry 136:424–426, 1979

Briere J, Zaidi LY: Sexual abuse histories and sequelae in female psychiatric emergency room patients. Am J Psychiatry 146:1602–1606, 1989

Frank H, Hoffman N: Borderline empathy: an empirical investigation. Compr Psychiatry 27:387–395, 1986

Frank H, Paris J: Recollections of family experience in borderline patients. Arch Gen Psychiatry 38:1031–1034, 1981

Goldberg RL, Mann LS, Wise TN, et al: Parental qualities as perceived by borderline personality disorders. Hillside Journal of Clinical Psychiatry 7:134–140, 1985

Grinker RR, Werble B, Drye RC: The Borderline Syndrome: A Behavioral Study of Ego-Functions. New York, Basic Books, 1968

Gunderson JG: Borderline Personality Disorder. Washington, DC, American Psychiatric Press, 1984

Gunderson J, Kerr J, Englund D: The families of borderlines: a comparative study. Arch Gen Psychiatry 37:27–33, 1980

Herman JL: Histories of violence in an outpatient population: an exploratory study. Am J Orthopsychiatry 56:137–141, 1986

Herman JL, van der Kolk BA: Traumatic antecedents of borderline personality disorder, in Psychological Trauma. Edited by van der Kolk BA. Washington, DC, American Psychiatric Press, 1987, pp 111–126

Herman JL, Perry JC, van der Kolk BA: Childhood trauma in borderline personality disorder. Am J Psychiatry 146:490–495, 1989

Kernberg O: Borderline Conditions and Pathological Narcissism. New York, Jason Aronson, 1975

Links PS, Steiner M, Offord DR, et al: Characteristics of borderline personality disorder: a Canadian study. Can J Psychiatry 33:336–340, 1988

Loftus EF: The reality of repressed memories. Am Psychol 48:518–537, 1993

Mahler M: A study of the separation-individuation process and its possible application to borderline phenomena in the psychoanalytic situation. Psychoanal Study Child 26:403–424, 1971

Masterson J: Treatment of the Borderline Adolescent: A Developmental Approach. New York, Wiley, 1972

Ogata SN, Silk KR, Goodrich S, et al: Childhood sexual and physical abuse in adult patients with borderline personality disorder. Am J Psychiatry 147:1008–1013, 1990

Paris J, Frank H: Perceptions of parental bonding in borderline patients. Am J Psychiatry 146:1498–1499, 1989

Pope HG Jr, Jonas JM, Hudson JI, et al: The validity of DSM-III borderline personality disorder. Arch Gen Psychiatry 40:23–30, 1983

Salzman JP, Salzman C, Wolfson AN, et al: Association between borderline personality structure and history of childhood abuse in adult volunteers. Compr Psychiatry 34:254–257, 1993

Shearer SL, Peters CP, Quaytman MS, et al: Frequency and correlates of childhood sexual and physical abuse histories in adult female borderline inpatients. Am J Psychiatry 147:214–216, 1990

Soloff PH, Millward JW: Developmental histories of borderline patients. Compr Psychiatry 24:574–588, 1983

Stern A: Psychoanalytic investigation of and therapy in the borderline group of neuroses. Psychoanal Q 7:467–489, 1938

Stone MH: The Borderline Syndromes: Constitution, Personality, and Adaptation. New York, McGraw-Hill, 1980

Walsh F: The family of the borderline patient, in The Borderline Patient. Edited by Grinker RR, Werble B. New York, Jason Aronson, 1977, pp 158–177

Wender PH: The contribution of the adoption studies to an understanding of the phenomenology and etiology of borderline schizophrenia, in Borderline Personality Disorders: The Concept, the Syndrome, the Patient. Edited by Hartocollis P. New York, International Universities Press, 1977, pp 255–269

Westen D, Ludolph P, Misle B, et al: Physical and sexual abuse in adolescent girls with borderline personality disorder. Am J Orthopsychiatry 60:55–66, 1990

Zanarini MC, Gunderson JG, Frankenburg FR, et al: Discriminating borderline personality disorder from other Axis II disorders. Am J Psychiatry 147:161–167, 1990

Zanarini MC: BPD as an impulse spectrum disorder, in Borderline Personality Disorder: Etiology and Treatment. Edited by Paris J. Washington, DC, American Psychiatric Press, 1993, pp 67–85

Chapter 2

Parameters of Childhood Sexual Abuse in Female Patients

Joel Paris, M.D., and Hallie Zweig-Frank, Ph.D.

Borderline patients have a high rate of reported childhood sexual abuse (CSA). Seven studies have confirmed this association (Byrne et al. 1990; Herman et al. 1989; Links et al. 1988; Ogata et al. 1990b; Shearer et al. 1990; Westen et al. 1990; Zanarini et al. 1989a). However, there are important unanswered questions about the nature of this relationship. To what extent can the trauma of sexual abuse in childhood account for the complex pathology seen in adults with borderline personality disorder (BPD)? Evidence from many studies that have examined the sequelae of a wide variety of childhood trauma suggests that single negative events of any kind do not on the whole have long-term psychological sequelae in adulthood (Rutter 1987, 1989). The exceptions involve trauma of a severe nature or traumas associated with other risk factors, leading to a cumulative effect (Rutter and Rutter 1993). Our research is in line with these other studies in that it was designed to examine histories of CSA in sufficient detail both to determine their severity and to examine to what extent the effects of sexual abuse can be accounted for by the presence of other risk factors during childhood.

To examine the severity of CSA, we developed a methodology based on the large number of community studies of the long-term effects of CSA. The discussion below follows a comprehen-

---

This study was supported by the National Health Research Development Program, Health and Welfare Canada, Grant 6605-3486-CSA.

sive review by Browne and Finkelhor (1986). Research reports indicate that a history of CSA is associated with a number of phenomena also characteristic of borderline patients: unstable mood, suicide attempts, substance abuse, problems in intimate relationships, and sexual revictimization. On the other hand, these studies also show that fewer than a quarter of those with a CSA history have any demonstrable long-term sequelae. The explanation seems to be that the presence of sequelae is highly dependent on the parameters of the abuse. These parameters include relationship to the perpetrator, frequency, duration, age at onset, nature of the abuse, use of force, disclosure, and whether help was obtained after disclosure. Of these, the most consistent predictors of long-term sequelae are a perpetrator who is a caretaker (especially in father-daughter incest), sexual acts of greater severity (especially penetration), and CSA of greater frequency and duration. Since a minority of CSA reports involve either incest or penetration, and since most are of single incidents, it is not surprising that CSA is generally followed by immediate but not necessarily long-term sequelae. Major psychopathology is most likely to develop when the parameters of sexual abuse are severe.

A limitation of the previous studies of CSA in borderline patients is that they have not examined these parameters of abuse in detail. In fact, many of these reports considered sexual abuse as a single variable. Four studies (Links et al. 1988; Ogata et al. 1990b; Westen et al. 1990; Zanarini et al. 1989a) did determine the relationship to the perpetrator. The samples in the seven studies were generally too small to examine all the other parameters. The first goal of the present study was, therefore, to examine in a large sample of borderline patients all the parameters of CSA that have been looked at in the community studies in order to determine whether, in addition to any overall relationship between CSA and BPD, any of these CSA parameters have a specific relationship with the borderline diagnosis.

Another limitation of the previous research on psychological risk factors for BPD is the use of univariate designs. Community studies have suggested that some of the effects of childhood sexual abuse are attributable to other psychological factors. For example, there have been two empirical studies using multivariate designs (Fromuth 1986; Nash et al. 1993) in which parental neglect accounted for the pathological effects of CSA. The other psychological risk factors shown to be associated with BPD need to be examined in the same study as measures of sexual abuse. These factors include significantly higher frequencies of intrafamilial physical abuse (Herman et al. 1989; Links et al. 1988), of separation from or loss of parents early in life (Bradley 1979; Links et al. 1988; Paris et al. 1988; Zanarini et al. 1989a), and of abnormal parental bonding in BPD (Goldberg et al. 1985; Torgersen and Alnaes 1992; Zweig-Frank and Paris 1991). It is important to determine whether the effects of CSA are related to BPD above and beyond these other factors. The examination of CSA and other psychological risk factors in multivariate analyses was, therefore, the second goal of the present study.

The most critical test of specificity for any risk factor for BPD is whether it discriminates borderline from nonborderline personality disorders. Therefore, in this study, borderline patients were compared with a group of patients who had other Axis II disorders. In this chapter we describe the findings of the first stage of the project, which was confined to female patients.

METHOD

Subjects

All subjects were female current or former patients between the ages of 18 and 48 who had been treated in the outpatient department of a university hospital. A research assistant searched chart records from the previous 2 years and identified 200 subjects who had received a diagnosis of a personality disorder, excluding any patients with diagnoses of schizophrenia, bipolar mood disorder, or organic brain syndrome. Of these, 174 agreed to enter the study with informed consent. Another 24 subjects of the 174 were eliminated by interview: 7 because they were found to have exclusion diagnoses, 13 because they had met criteria for BPD in the past but had recovered from the disorder, and 4 because they had equivocal scores on the main diagnostic instrument and could not be clearly assigned to BPD or non-BPD groups.

The final sample consisted of 150 patients, of whom 78 were in the BPD group and 72 were in the non-BPD group. The mean age for the BPD group was 28.3 (SD = 6.3) and for the non-BPD group, 29.7 (SD = 7.2, t = –1.3, df = 148, NS). There were differences in both marital status and education between the groups; the borderline patients were less likely to be married (χ^2 = 11.5, df = 4, P = .02) and had less education ($\chi2$ = 14.5, df = 4, P < .02) than the non-BPD group.

Diagnoses on Axis II were made for the non-BPD subjects by the interviewing psychiatrist (J.P.), using the Diagnostic Interview for Personality Disorders (DIPD; Zanarini et al. 1987). The distribution was as follows: 4 in the DSM-criteria cluster A of personality disorders (1 paranoid, 3 schizotypal), 8 in cluster B (all histrionic), and 27 in cluster C (13 dependent, 9 avoidant, 3 compulsive, 2 passive-aggressive). There were 33 additional patients who did not meet criteria for any specific disorder but who met DSM-III-R criteria for personality disorder not otherwise specified (American Psychiatric Association 1987).

Measures

Diagnosis

Assignment to the BPD or non-BPD groups was determined by using the Revised Diagnostic Interview for Borderlines (Zanarini et al. 1989b), a well-validated semistructured interview for separating borderline from nonborderline personality disorders, which uses the recommended cutoff of 8 out of 10 for a positive diagnosis of BPD. All interviews were carried out by a psychiatrist who had extensive experience with the instrument (J.P.). A reliability check was also carried out with a second psychiatrist on a subsample of 10 borderline and 10 nonborderline subjects, and the kappa for diagnostic agreement was .90.

Developmental Interview

This semistructured interview was used to score histories of CSA and its parameters, physical abuse and its parameters, and separation or loss. It consists of a wide range of questions about childhood development in which the items about abuse are embedded. Most of the questions were derived from two previous instruments used for this purpose (Herman et al. 1989; Ogata et al. 1990a). The developmental interview was conducted by an experienced psychiatrist who was blind to diagnosis, and it lasted about 2 hours.

As part of the developmental interview, each subject was questioned about memories of abuse occurring during the first 16 years of her life. Sexual abuse was defined as unwanted sexual contact, ranging from fondling to sexual intercourse, initiated by someone 5 or more years older or by a family member. The presence of CSA was scored dichotomously. When abuse was reported to have occurred, separate questions were asked about each parameter. Perpetrators were classified as father, mother, stepfather, stepmother, sibling, other relative, nonrelative, or stranger. If more than one person was reported, the subject was scored as having multiple perpetrators. Frequency was recorded on a 5-point scale, ranging from a single incident to very often. Duration was recorded in number of months. Age at onset was recorded in years. Nature of abuse was recorded by separately scoring four types: fondling, genital fondling, oral sex, and penetration. The presence of force, the ability to disclose the abuse at the time, and the success of attempts to get help were all scored dichotomously.

Physical abuse was scored dichotomously. Its presence was recorded only if the perpetrator was a caretaker.

Separation or loss was scored if there was any death or permanent separation from a parent any time in the first 16 years of life, and it was scored separately if occurring only in the first 5 years of life.

Parental Bonding Index

A well-known 25-item self-report measure, the Parental Bonding Index (PBI), was used for recollections of affection and control from each parent over the first 16 years of life (Parker 1983). Subjects score their perceptions of parental behavior on a 4-point

Likert scale (0–3) applied to 12 items concerning affection (range 0–36) and 13 items concerning control (range 0–39).

RESULTS

CSA and Its Parameters

The overall rate of CSA was 70.5% (55 subjects) in the BPD sample and 45.8% (33) in the non-BPD sample. This difference was highly significant ($\chi^2 = 9.4$, df = 1, $P < .002$).

The rates of CSA were examined separately for each type of perpetrator in the two diagnostic groups (Table 2–1). There were no significant differences between the groups for any caretaker (father, mother, stepfather, stepmother). The overall rate for caretaker abuse was 29.5% (23) in the BPD group and 36.1% (26) in the non-BPD group. This difference was not significant. The difference in the frequency of overall CSA between the diagnostic groups was accounted for by higher rates from the following perpetrators: siblings ($\chi^2 = 4.4$, df = 1, $P < .05$), other relatives

Table 2–1. Rates of childhood sexual abuse in borderline and nonborderline patients by perpetrator

Perpetrator	BPD (%) (n = 78)	non-BPD (%) (n = 72)
Overall***	70.5	45.8
Father	14.1	15.3
Mother	5.1	1.4
Stepfather	5.1	2.8
Stepmother	1.3	0.0
Siblings*	14.1	4.2
Other relatives**	24.4	8.3
Nonrelatives**	34.6	15.3
Strangers	19.2	15.3
Any caretaker	29.5	36.1
Multiple***	37.2	13.9

*$P < .05$. **$P < .01$. ***$P < .002$.

(χ^2 = 6.9, df = 1, P < .01), and nonrelatives (χ^2 = 7.4, df = 1, P < .01). The frequency of multiple perpetrators was also significantly higher in the BPD group (37.2%; 29) than in the non-BPD group (13.9%; 10) (χ^2 = 10.6, df = 1, P < .002). The subjects from both diagnostic groups who reported CSA were compared with respect to all the parameters of sexual abuse (Table 2–2). Continuous variables were analyzed by t tests and dichotomous variables by χ^2 tests. Because a large number of abused subjects had been abused by more than one perpetrator, the data were entered for the perpetrator whose abuse would be expected to be more traumatic, according to the following hierarchy: father, mother, stepfather, stepmother, sibling, other relative, nonrelative, stranger.

There were no differences between the abused BPD and non-BPD groups with respect to the parameters of frequency or duration. The distributions of both CSA frequency and du-

Table 2–2. Parameters of childhood sexual abuse in borderline and nonborderline personality disorders

Parameter	BPD (n = 55)	non-BPD (n = 33)
Frequency (%)		
Single incident	80.0	66.7
Rarely	0.0	9.1
Sometimes	0.0	3.0
Often	16.4	18.2
Very often	3.6	3.0
Duration (months)	26.5	27.5
Age at onset (years)	9.0	9.2
Nature (%)		
Fondling	84.3	93.1
Genital fondling	74.5	57.6
Oral sex	20.0	9.1
Penetration*	32.7	6.1
Force (%)	92.7	90.9
Disclosure (%)	30.9	36.4
Help (%)	16.4	15.2

*P < .005.

ration in the BPD group were bimodal: the largest number of CSA reports from borderline subjects described single incidents and short duration, whereas a smaller but substantial number of CSA reports from borderline subjects described CSA as frequent and with a duration of years. There were no significant differences between the abused groups for age at onset, force, disclosure, or help. There was, however, a large significant difference between the groups with respect to the nature of their CSA. Although the two abused groups did not differ significantly in the prevalence of fondling, genital fondling, or oral sex, there was a highly significant difference for prevalence of penetration, which occurred in 32.7% (18) of the abused BPD group and 6.1% (2) of the abused non-BPD group (χ^2 = 8.4, df = 1, P < .004). The subjects with histories of penetration were also significantly more likely to have been abused by multiple perpetrators (χ^2 = 5.3, df = 1, P < .02).

To examine whether any of the parameters of sexual abuse were able to discriminate the two diagnostic groups much better than the others, a logistic regression of the CSA parameters on diagnosis was carried out in all subjects who reported CSA. The only significant variable was penetration (β = .84, P < .05, odds ratio 2.3).

Physical Abuse, Separation or Loss, and Parental Bonding

There was a significant difference between the two groups in the overall rate of physical abuse, which was 73.1% (57) for the BPD group and 52.8% (38) for the non-BPD group (χ^2 = 6.6, df = 1, P < .05). The overall rate of separation from or loss of a parent at any time before the age of 16 was 51.3% (40) for the BPD group and 45.8% (33) for the non-BPD group. The rate before the age of 5 was 21.8% (17) for the BPD group and 13.9% (10) for the non-BPD group. Neither of these differences was significant. A comparison of the mean scores on the four PBI scales showed a significant difference between the BPD and non-BPD groups only on the maternal affection scale; the borderline group had a lower score on this measure (t = −2.0, df = 148, P < .05).

Multivariate Analysis

A logistic regression was carried out; the independent variables were sexual abuse, physical abuse, the four PBI scores, and separation or loss before the age of 16. The only significant variable in the regression was sexual abuse ($\beta = .47$, $P < .02$, odds ratio 1.6). The two other variables that had been significant in the univariate analyses (physical abuse and maternal affection) no longer attained significance in the multivariate analysis.

DISCUSSION

Our findings support the large number of studies showing that histories of CSA are particularly common in patients with BPD. However, the overlap between the BPD and non-BPD groups was large: not all borderline subjects reported abuse, and nearly half of the nonborderline subjects did.

By examining the parameters of CSA, we aimed to discriminate BPD from non-BPD cases with more precision. When we took into consideration relationship to perpetrator, the rate of CSA in BPD from caretakers alone was only 29%, compared to 71% when all categories of perpetrators were combined. These percentages closely parallel the results of two other studies (Links et al. 1988; Zanarini et al. 1989a). In contrast to one earlier report (Westen et al. 1990), in which incest histories were found to be frequent in an inpatient sample of borderline adolescents, fewer than 20% of subjects in either group reported father-daughter or stepfather-stepdaughter incest. The difference in the overall rates of CSA between our two groups was accounted for by an increased frequency of abuse in the BPD group from siblings, from other relatives, and from nonrelatives. This distribution is virtually identical to that of an earlier report (Ogata et al. 1990b). The higher frequency of multiple perpetrators in the BPD group also confirms findings reported by Ogata et al. This result suggests that the cumulative effects of revictimization could be a risk factor in its own right for BPD.

The two groups did not differ with respect to the majority of the other parameters of CSA. It is notable that, as in the community studies, most of the reports of CSA in both groups were of single incidents. The one parameter that did discriminate abused BPD and non-BPD subjects was the nature of sexual abuse. CSA with penetration was found significantly more frequently in the borderline group in univariate analysis, and penetration was also the only parameter that discriminated between the two diagnostic groups in multivariate analysis. In fact, if one were to exclude from the analysis the subjects who reported CSA with penetration, the overall rates of sexual abuse in the borderline and nonborderline samples would be virtually identical. These findings have a parallel in the results of multivariate community studies, which found that penetration was the single most powerful predictor of psychopathology in adults with CSA (Peters 1988; Russell 1986). Our other findings did not correspond to the findings of other community studies, in which duration (Briere 1988) or the use of force (Finkelhor 1979) were powerful predictors of psychopathology.

In relation to the question whether CSA has an effect independent of other risk factors, the multivariate analysis showed that only a history of CSA discriminated borderline from nonborderline personality disorders more than the other psychological factors measured here. Very similar findings have been reported in two other studies (Links and van Reekum 1993; Ogata et al. 1990b). However, these results stand in contrast to those reported by Zanarini et al. (Chapter 3, this volume).

The results could to some extent be interpreted as being consistent with the hypothesis that the traumatic effects of sexual abuse on children can lead to borderline psychopathology (Herman and van der Kolk 1987). Not only was CSA more common in BPD, but the parameters of CSA severity increased discrimination between the groups. Finally, there was no evidence that these effects were secondary to other psychological factors.

Several other findings, however, are not consistent with a posttraumatic hypothesis. First, there was a great overlap in rates of CSA between the borderline subjects and the Axis II control subjects. Second, the majority of the parameters failed to discriminate between the groups. Third, the two measures of severity (penetration and multiple perpetrators) that did discriminate between the groups were reported to have occurred only by a minority of the borderline patients. Finally, there was a preponderance of single incidents among the reports of CSA even in the borderline group. What the results in fact seem to suggest is that there may be a subgroup of patients with BPD in which CSA plays a particularly important role. In that subgroup of patients (about a quarter of our borderline sample), severe CSA discriminated borderline from nonborderline patients more strongly. However, in the majority of BPD cases, CSA either lacked the parameters of severity (penetration and multiple perpetrators) or was absent.

In the patients with severe CSA, the precise mechanism by which trauma increases the risk for BPD remains to be elucidated. In addition to the direct effects of trauma, sexual abuse during childhood has important effects on cognition and self-esteem (Finkelhor 1988). It would be premature to consider BPD, as some have suggested (Herman and van der Kolk 1987), a chronic posttraumatic stress disorder.

It is also possible that there are psychological risk factors other than those that we examined that could influence whether CSA leads to BPD. For example, our measure of family pathology, the PBI, is not very specific for any psychiatric diagnosis (Parker 1983). We might have found different results if we had used measures of family structure, which have been shown to be abnormal in BPD (Ogata et al. 1990a). Another important possibility involves the interaction of trauma with biological risk factors. Although no specific biological markers have been found for BPD (van Reekum et al. 1993), Siever and Davis (1991) have hypothesized that there are underlying personality dimensions (affective instability and impulsivity) that are necessary conditions for BPD and that are under genetic control.

The limitations of this study are associated with the problems of retrospective self-report. It is possible that borderline patients, who suffer from distorted perceptions of the world, may be particularly susceptible to false memories (Loftus 1979). But none of our subjects had repressed memories of abuse that emerged only from psychotherapy.

The picture of a traumatic childhood reported by borderline patients has been consistent in many studies with different methodologies. Moreover, the more detailed picture of CSA in this study, obtained by examining all the parameters of abuse, suggests greater validity for our results. Finally, empirical studies of childhood memories in psychiatric patients have shown that the more concrete the event, the more verifiable it is (Robins et al. 1985). It has been shown that reports of some forms of CSA, such as incest, can be verified through sibling concordance (Herman and Schatzow 1987).

In summary, our findings are consistent with other reports of a greater prevalence of sexual abuse in BPD and have provided confirmation in a larger sample. That the association between CSA and BPD may have etiological significance is suggested by its independent effect in multivariate analysis. However, the analysis of the parameters of CSA suggests that this relationship is most important for a subgroup of borderline patients who have had more severe trauma during childhood.

REFERENCES

American Psychiatric Association: Diagnostic and Statistical Manual of Mental Disorders, 3rd Edition, Revised. Washington, DC, American Psychiatric Association, 1987

Bradley SJ: The relationship of early maternal separation to borderline personality in children and adolescents: a pilot study. Am J Psychiatry 136:424–426, 1979

Briere J: The long-term clinical correlates of childhood sexual victimization. Ann N Y Acad Sci 528:327–334, 1988

Browne A, Finkelhor D: Impact of child sexual abuse: a review of the research. Psychol Bull 99:66–77, 1986

Byrne CP, Velamoor VR, Cernovsky ZZ, et al: a comparison of borderline and schizophrenic patients for childhood life events and parent-child relationships. Can J Psychiatry 35:590–595, 1990

Finkelhor D: Sexually Victimized Children. New York, Free Press, 1979

Finkelhor D: The trauma of child sexual abuse: two models, in Lasting Effects of Child Sexual Abuse. Edited by Wyatt GE, Powell GJ. Beverly Hills, CA, Sage, 1988, pp 61–82

Fromuth ME: The relationship of childhood sexual abuse with later psychological and sexual adjustment in a sample of college women. Child Abuse Negl 10:5–15, 1986

Goldberg RL, Mann LS, Wise TN, et al: Parental qualities as perceived by borderline personality disorders. Hillside Journal of Clinical Psychiatry 7:134–140, 1985

Herman JL, Schatzow E: Recovery and verification of memories of childhood sexual trauma. Psychoanalytic Psychology 4:1–14, 1987

Herman JL, van der Kolk BA: Traumatic antecedents of borderline personality disorder, in Psychological Trauma. Edited by van der Kolk BA. Washington, DC, American Psychiatric Press, 1987, pp 111–126

Herman JL, Perry JC, van der Kolk BA: Childhood trauma in borderline personality disorder. Am J Psychiatry 146:490–495, 1989

Links PS, van Reekum R: Childhood sexual abuse, parental impairment and the development of borderline personality disorder. Can J Psychiatry 38:472–474, 1993

Links PS, Steiner M, Offord DR, et al: Characteristics of borderline personality disorder: a Canadian study. Can J Psychiatry 33:336–340, 1988

Loftus E: Eyewitness Testimony. Cambridge, MA, Harvard University Press, 1979

Nash MR, Hulsey TL, Sexton MC, et al: Long-term sequelae of childhood sexual abuse: perceived family environment, psychopathology, and dissociation. J Consult Clin Psychol 61:276–283, 1993

Ogata SN, Silk KR, Goodrich S: The childhood experience of the borderline patient, in Family Environment and Borderline Personality Disorder. Edited by Links PS. Washington, DC, American Psychiatric Press, 1990a, pp 87–103

Ogata SN, Silk KR, Goodrich S, et al: Childhood sexual and physical abuse in adult patients with borderline personality disorder. Am J Psychiatry 147:1008–1013, 1990b

Paris J, Nowlis D, Brown R: Developmental factors in the outcome of borderline personality disorder. Compr Psychiatry 29:147–150, 1988;

Parker G: Parental Overprotection: a Risk Factor in Psychosocial Development. New York, Grune & Stratton, 1983

Peters SD: Child sexual abuse and later psychological problems, in Lasting Effects of Child Sexual Abuse. Edited by Wyatt GE, Powell GJ. Beverly Hills, CA, Sage, 1988, pp 101–117

Robins LN, Schoenberg SP, Holmes SJ, et al: Early home environment and retrospective recall: a test for concordance between siblings with and without psychiatric disorders. Am J Orthopsychiatry 55:27–41, 1985

Russell DEH: The Secret Trauma: Incest in the Lives of Girls and Women. New York, Basic Books, 1986

Rutter M: Psychosocial resilience and protective mechanisms. Am J Orthopsychiatry 57:316–331, 1987

Rutter M: Pathways from childhood to adult life. J Child Psychol Psychiatry 30:23–51, 1989

Rutter M, Rutter M: Developing Minds: Challenge and Continuity Across the Life Span. New York, Basic Books, 1993

Shearer SL, Peters CP, Quaytman MS, et al: Frequency and correlates of childhood sexual and physical abuse histories in adult female borderline inpatients. Am J Psychiatry 147:214–216, 1990

Siever LJ, Davis KL: a psychobiological perspective on the personality disorders. Am J Psychiatry 148:1647–1658, 1991

Torgersen S, Alnaes R: Differential perception of parental bonding in schizotypal and borderline personality disorder patients. Compr Psychiatry 33:34–38, 1992

van Reekum R, Links PS, Boiago I: Constitutional factors in borderline personality disorder: genetics, brain dysfunction, and biological markers, in Borderline Personality Disorder: Etiology and Treatment. Edited by Paris J. Washington, DC, American Psychiatric Press, 1993, pp 13–38

Westen D, Ludolph P, Misle B, et al: Physical and sexual abuse in adolescent girls with borderline personality disorder. Am J Orthopsychiatry 60:55–66, 1990

Zanarini MC, Frankenburg FR, Chauncey DL, et al: The Diagnostic Interview for Personality Disorders: interrater and test-retest reliability. Compr Psychiatry 28:467–480, 1987

Zanarini MC, Gunderson JG, Marino MF, et al: Childhood experiences of borderline patients. Compr Psychiatry 30:18–25, 1989a

Zanarini MC, Gunderson JG, Frankenburg FR, et al: The Revised Diagnostic Interview for Borderlines: discriminating BPD from other Axis II disorders. J Personality Disorders 3:10–18, 1989b

Zweig-Frank H, Paris J: Parents' emotional neglect and overprotection according to the recollections of patients with borderline personality disorder. Am J Psychiatry 148:648–651, 1991

Chapter 3

Childhood Factors Associated With the Development of Borderline Personality Disorder

Mary C. Zanarini, Ed.D., Elyse D. Dubo, M.D., F.R.C.P.(C.), Ruth E. Lewis, Ph.D., and Amy A. Williams, B.S.

Initial studies of the childhood experiences of patients with borderline personality disorder (BPD) focused on the etiological role of early separations (Akiskal et al. 1985; Bradley 1979; Soloff and Millward 1983; Walsh 1977) and relatively subtle forms of neglect (Frank and Hoffman 1986; Frank and Paris 1981; Goldberg et al. 1985; Grinker et al. 1968; Gunderson et al. 1980; Paris and Frank 1989; Soloff and Millward 1983; Walsh 1977). However, more recent studies have focused on the role of childhood abuse in the etiology of BPD (Herman et al. 1989; Links et al. 1988; Ogata et al. 1990; Salzman et al. 1993; Shearer et al. 1990; Westen et al. 1990; Zanarini et al. 1989a).

These studies found that both physical and sexual abuse are commonly reported by borderline patients. More specifically, these studies have found that 10%–71% of borderline patients report having been physically abused by a parent or other adult caretaker (Herman et al. 1989; Links et al. 1988; Ogata et al. 1990; Salzman et al. 1993; Shearer et al. 1990; Westen et al. 1990; Zanarini et al. 1989a) and that 0%–33% report having had an incestuous relationship with a full-time adult caretaker (Links et al. 1988; Ogata et al. 1990; Salzman et al. 1993; Shearer et al. 1990; Westen et al. 1990; Zanarini et al. 1989a). The studies that also

Supported in part by National Institute of Mental Health grant MH47588.

investigated the prevalence of childhood sexual abuse by non-caretakers found that overall rates of childhood sexual abuse reported by borderline patients ranged from 16% to 71% (Herman et al. 1989; Ogata et al. 1990; Salzman et al. 1993; Shearer et al. 1990; Westen et al. 1990).

Although most of the relevant studies found that a childhood history of physical abuse was commonly reported by borderline patients, only one found that it is discriminating (Links et al. 1988). In contrast, all the relevant studies found that a significantly higher percentage of borderline patients than of control subjects with near-neighbor disorders (depression, other forms of personality disorder) reported a childhood history of sexual abuse (Herman et al. 1989; Links et al. 1988; Ogata et al. 1990; Westen et al. 1990; Zanarini et al. 1989a).

The latter results were interpreted by some to mean that sexual abuse is the main etiological factor in the development of BPD (Herman and van der Kolk 1987). They were also interpreted to mean that patients meeting current criteria for BPD might be better conceptualized as having a chronic form of post-traumatic stress disorder (PTSD) than as having BPD (Herman 1992; Herman and van der Kolk 1987).

In the research reported in this chapter, we placed in perspective the role of childhood sexual abuse in the etiology of BPD by studying a wide range of pathological childhood experiences in a sample of 78 patients with criteria-defined BPD and 37 control subjects with other Axis II disorders. The study improved on the design of earlier studies through the relatively large size of the patient groups, the rigor with which the patients were diagnosed, and the fact that—unlike all previous studies—the study assessed numerous forms of pathological childhood experiences blind to diagnostic status. The study also improved on the design of most earlier studies by using multivariate analyses to assess the relative contributions of these childhood factors.

METHOD

This study began as one site of the DSM-IV Axis II Field Trials but evolved into a larger study of the validity of BPD. Briefly,

115 inpatients at McLean Hospital in Belmont, Massachusetts, were interviewed about all aspects of their phenomenology as well as their family history of psychiatric disorder and pathological childhood experiences.

More specifically, each patient was initially screened to determine that he or she 1) was between the ages of 18 and 60, 2) had normal or better intelligence, 3) had no history or current symptomatology of a serious organic condition or major psychotic disorder (e.g., schizophrenia or bipolar disorder), and 4) had been given a definite or probable Axis II diagnosis by the admitting physician. Written informed consent was obtained from each patient. Three semistructured diagnostic interviews were then administered to each patient by one of four diagnosticians: a board-certified psychiatrist, one of two senior psychiatric residents, or a clinically experienced bachelor's-level research assistant. All four diagnosticians had been trained in the administration and scoring of these instruments by the senior author (M.C.Z.), and adequate levels of interrater reliability had been obtained during this training period.

The following instruments were administered to each patient, blind to his or her clinical diagnosis: 1) the Structured Clinical Interview for DSM-III-R Axis I Disorders (SCID-I), which included a PTSD module devised at McLean (Spitzer et al. 1990), 2) the Revised Diagnostic Interview for Borderlines (DIB-R)—a semistructured interview that can reliably distinguish clinically diagnosed borderline patients from those with other Axis II disorders (Zanarini et al. 1989b), and 3) the Revised Diagnostic Interview for Personality Disorders (DIPD-R)— a semistructured interview that reliably assesses the presence of the 13 Axis II disorders described in DSM-III-R (Zanarini et al. 1987).

Information concerning pathological childhood experiences was assessed by one of two clinically experienced research assistants, each of whom was blind to all other data concerning each patient, including his or her current diagnostic status. Pathological childhood experiences were assessed with the Revised Childhood Experiences Questionnaire, a semistructured interview whose psychometric properties have been described elsewhere (Zanarini et al. 1989a). Briefly, this instrument inquires about

4 forms of abuse and 7 forms of neglect engaged in by full-time caretakers, sexual abuse by noncaretakers, and 12 types of separations from full-time caretakers that lasted 1 month or more. For an item to be given a positive rating, detailed information concerning the event in question had to be provided.

RESULTS

All told, 78 patients met both DIB-R and DSM-III-R criteria for BPD, and another 37 met DSM-III-R criteria for at least one nonborderline Axis II disorder. Twelve of the 37 control subjects (32.4%) met DSM-III-R criteria for a very-near-neighbor Axis II disorder, antisocial personality disorder.

Demographically, borderline patients and Axis II control subjects were found to be similar in mean age (30.0 ± 9.5 vs. 33.6 ± 9.5 years). However, a significantly higher percentage of borderline patients (67.9%, or 53) than control subjects (40.5%, or 15) were female. In addition, borderline patients, on average, came from a significantly lower socioeconomic background (although still middle class) than the background of Axis II control subjects, as measured by the 5-point (1 = highest, 5 = lowest) Hollingshead-Redlich scale (3.2 ± 1.1 vs. 2.7 ± 1.2).

Table 3–1 compares the borderline patients and the Axis II control subjects on reported rates of abuse and neglect. At the .05 level of significance or greater, a significantly higher percentage of borderline patients than of control subjects reported a childhood history of physical abuse, sexual abuse by noncaretakers, overall sexual abuse, emotional withdrawal by a caretaker, and lack of a real relationship with a caretaker. (Because these and subsequent univariate analyses were hypothesis driven and confirmed prior research findings, the Bonferroni Correction for Multiple Comparisons was not used.)

About equal percentages of borderline patients (21.8%, or 17 patients) and control subjects (24.3%, or 9 subjects) reported having experienced a prolonged separation from a caretaker before the age of 6. The mean number of early childhood separations reported by borderline patients ($.46 \pm 1.1$) and control subjects ($.49 \pm 1.3$) was also basically the same.

Table 3–1. Pathological childhood experiences of borderline patients and Axis II control subjects

Experience	Borderline (%)	Other PD (%)
Emotional abuse	75.6	64.9
Verbal abuse	79.5	70.3
Physical abuse	60.3	32.4**
Caretaker sexual abuse	29.5	18.9
Noncaretaker sexual abuse	53.8	21.6**
Any sexual abuse	59.0	35.1*
Any abuse	91.0	81.1
Physical neglect	21.8	10.8
Emotional withdrawal	61.5	35.1*
Inconsistent treatment	50.0	37.8
Denial of feelings	65.4	51.4
Lack of a real relationship	83.3	64.9*
Parentification of patient	51.3	37.8
Failure to provide protection	42.3	35.1
Any neglect	93.6	86.5

*P .05. **P < .01. (P levels are from corrected χ^2 analyses.)

Table 3–2 compares the rates of abuse and neglect reported by the 46 borderline patients with a childhood history of sexual abuse and the 32 without such a childhood history. At the.05 level of significance or greater, a significantly higher percentage of sexually abused than non–sexually-abused borderline patients reported a childhood history of emotional abuse, physical abuse, any abuse, emotional withdrawal, and failure by a caretaker to provide needed protection.

A slightly higher percentage of sexually abused borderline patients (26.1%, or 12) than nonabused borderline patients (15.6%, or 5) reported having experienced a prolonged separation from a caretaker before the age of 6. The mean number of early-childhood separations reported by sexually abused borderline patients (0.61 ± 1.4) was also slightly but not significantly higher than that reported by non–sexually-abused borderline patients (0.25 ± 6.7).

Table 3-2. Pathological childhood experiences of borderline patients who were and were not sexually abused

Experience	Sexually abused (%) (n = 46)	Not sexually abused (%) (n = 32)
Emotional abuse	89.1	56.3**
Verbal abuse	87.0	68.8
Physical abuse	71.7	43.8*
Any abuse	97.8	78.1**
Physical neglect	26.1	15.6
Emotional withdrawal	78.3	37.5***
Inconsistent treatment	56.5	40.6
Denial of feelings	65.2	65.6
Lack of a real relationship	87.0	78.1
Parentification of patient	54.3	46.9
Failure to provide protection	54.3	25.0*
Any neglect	95.7	90.6

*$P < .05$. **$P < .01$. ***$P < .001$. (P levels are from corrected χ^2 analyses.

These numerous univariate analyses reveal that sexual abuse almost always occurred in conjunction with at least one other type of abuse and/or neglect. A forced-entry logistic regression with diagnostic status (BPD vs. other PD) as the dependent variable was conducted next to determine the relative importance of these numerous pathological childhood experiences. A total of 25 independent variables were studied: patient gender and each of the abuse and neglect variables broken down by gender of the caretaker (or in the case of noncaretaker sexual abuse, the gender of the noncaretaker).

Five factors were significantly associated with an adult diagnosis of BPD (Table 3–3): being female, a childhood history of sexual abuse by a male caretaker, a childhood history of sexual abuse by a male noncaretaker, emotional withdrawal by a male caretaker, and lack of a real emotional relationship with a female caretaker. A patient who had experienced sexual abuse by a male caretaker had a risk of being diagnosed as having BPD that was about three times greater than that of a patient who did not report having had this childhood experience. A patient who had

Table 3–3. Significant risk factors associated with diagnosis of borderline personality disorder (BPD)[a]

Variable	P	Odds ratio
Female gender	.04	1.9
Sexual abuse by male caretaker	.02	3.0
Sexual abuse by male noncaretaker	.02	2.2
Emotional withdrawal by male caretaker	.03	2.1
Lack of real relationship with female caretaker	.04	2.1

[a]Forced-entry logistic regression with diagnosis (BPD/non-BPD) as dependent variable.

experienced the other four variables had a risk of being diagnosed as having BPD that was about two times greater than the risk for a patient who was male or who did not report having had these childhood experiences.

Concerns arose about the large number of independent variables used in the logistic regression described here and about the possible problem of multicolinearity. As a result, another forced-entry logistic regression was performed; it contained only variables that had achieved significance in between-group comparisons of borderline patients and control subjects: patient gender, physical abuse by a caretaker, overall sexual abuse, emotional withdrawal by a caretaker, and lack of a real emotional relationship with a caretaker. These childhood variables were entered by gender of caretaker, or, in the case of sexual abuse, by caretaker and/or noncaretaker. Thus, nine independent variables were entered into this logistic regression. Basically the same variables already found significant in the first logistic regression were also found in the second one to be significant risk factors for BPD: being female, a childhood history of sexual abuse by a male caretaker and/or a male noncaretaker, emotional withdrawal by a male caretaker, and lack of a real emotional relationship with a female caretaker. In terms of the these four variables, a patient's risk of being diagnosed as having BPD was about two times greater than that of a patient who was male or who did not report having had these childhood experiences.

DISCUSSION

Four important results emerged from this study. First, we found that childhood experiences of both abuse and neglect were basically ubiquitous for our borderline patients. More specifically, we found that 91% of our borderline patients reported some type of childhood abuse and that 94% reported some type of childhood neglect. In terms of specific forms of abuse, almost 80% of our borderline patients reported a childhood history of emotional or verbal abuse, and about 60% reported a childhood history of physical or sexual abuse. In terms of specific forms of neglect, more than 80% of our borderline patients reported that they lacked a real emotional relationship with one or more caretakers; about 60% reported a caretaker's withdrawing from them emotionally and a caretaker's denying their thoughts or feelings; about half reported being treated inconsistently, being parentified, and a caretaker's failing to provide them with needed protection; about a quarter reported being physically neglected during childhood.

The results of this study are consistent with those of earlier studies finding that a high percentage of borderline patients reported having been abused and/or neglected during childhood (Herman et al. 1989; Links et al. 1988; Ogata et al. 1990; Salzman et al. 1993; Shearer et al. 1990; Westen et al. 1990; Zanarini et al. 1989a). In terms of sexual abuse, we found that 29.5% (23) of our borderline patients reported being sexually abused by a caretaker during childhood. This rate falls within the range of rates (25%–33%) reported by most of the studies assessing the prevalence of this type of childhood experience (Links et al. 1988; Ogata et al. 1990; Shearer et al. 1990; Westen et al. 1990; Zanarini et al. 1989a). We also found an overall rate of childhood sexual abuse of 59% (46 patients). This rate is very consistent with the rates (40%–71%) reported for most other groups of borderline patients (Herman et al. 1989; Ogata et al. 1990; Shearer et al. 1990; Westen et al. 1990). The rates of caretaker and overall sexual abuse that we found are much higher than the rates (0%–16%) reported by Salzman et al. (1993). However, these differences are not surprising, because we were studying severely impaired inpatients, whereas Salzman et al. were studying symptomatic volunteers who had never been hospitalized for psychiatric reasons and who had not been self-destructive or suicidal for 4 years before entry into the study.

The second major finding of this study was that childhood experiences of both abuse and neglect were significantly more common among borderline patients than among control subjects. More specifically, physical abuse, sexual abuse by noncaretakers, overall sexual abuse, emotional withdrawal by a caretaker, and a lack of a real relationship with a caretaker were reported by a significantly higher percentage of borderline patients than control subjects. The results of this study are consistent with those of earlier studies finding that childhood experiences of both abuse and neglect are reported by a significantly higher percentage of borderline patients than of control subjects (Links et al. 1988; Westen et al. 1990; Zanarini et al. 1989a).

The third major finding of this study was that sexually abused borderline patients seemed to come from more chaotic environments than did non–sexually-abused borderline patients. They were significantly more likely than non–sexually-abused borderline patients to report having been emotionally abused, physically abused, abused in some nonsexual way, having a caretaker withdraw from them emotionally, and having a caretaker fail to provide them with needed protection. This, to the best of our knowledge, represents a new finding. It also emphasizes that sexual abuse does not occur in a vacuum but in a context of ongoing experiences of abuse and neglect.

The fourth major finding of this study is that when all types of pathological childhood experiences were considered together, sexual abuse seemed to be an important factor in the etiology of BPD, but that other factors, particularly neglect by caretakers of both genders, also played an important role. This, too, to the best of our knowledge, represents a new finding. It also underscores the fact that the development of BPD seems linked to the lack of optimal parenting by caretakers of both genders.

This finding concerning biparental neglect and sexual abuse makes intuitive clinical sense. It may be that biparental neglect puts the preborderline child at risk for being sexually abused by making it clear to potential perpetrators that no one will notice or care whether the child is abused. Biparental neglect may also put the preborderline child at risk for being sexually abused by leaving him or her with a strong unmet need for attention, care, and closeness that may be misinterpreted and/or manipulated by unscrupulous, sexually predatory individuals.

The results of this study are consistent with a multifactorial model of the etiology of BPD that we believe best captures the complexity of borderline psychopathology (Zanarini and Weinberg 1996). This model suggests that borderline symptomatology and its comorbid manifestations are the end product of a complex admixture of innate temperament, difficult childhood experiences, and relatively subtle forms of neurological and biochemical dysfunction (which may be sequelae of these childhood experiences or innate vulnerabilities).

This model is supported by recent research results that have found that BPD is associated with a temperament characterized by a high degree of neuroticism (i.e., emotional pain) as well as a low degree of agreeableness (i.e., strong individuality) (Clarkin et al. 1993; Soldz et al. 1993; Trull 1992). This model is also supported by recent research results that have found that subtle forms of neurological and biochemical dysfunction are common in borderline patients. More specifically, a series of studies have found that borderline patients often suffer from difficult-to-diagnose forms of neurological dysfunction (see Zanarini et al. 1994 for a review of studies in this area). In addition, biochemical studies have typically found low levels of serotonin in patients with problematic impulsivity, including criteria-defined borderline patients (Coccaro et al. 1989).

All these research findings suggest that painful childhood experiences join an extremely sensitive, tenacious temperament and subtle forms of biological dysfunction in the development of BPD. The exact relationship between these contributing factors is yet to be determined. It is also unclear whether these factors apply equally to all borderline patients or whether there are distinct subgroups of borderline patients.

Although these findings are still preliminary, they suggest a complex etiology for BPD that may include but not be limited to a childhood history of sexual abuse. Despite the robustness of these findings and their resonance with clinical experience over time with a variety of borderline patients, a relatively small group of clinicians refuse to believe most accounts of childhood sexual abuse, no matter how spontaneous, richly detailed, and affectively compelling the account. These clinicians often ask patients for corroborating evidence, despite the difficulty of obtaining such evidence and despite the fact that self-reports are the basic material of psychotherapy. Clearly, this type of behavior is demoralizing to borderline patients, who have often had a lifetime of having their feelings and experiences denied by those on whom they depend the most.

The evidence suggesting a complex etiology for BPD is also strenuously ignored by the clinicians who believe that sexual abuse per se is both a necessary and a sufficient precondition for the development of BPD. Although appealing in its simplicity, this view is simply not consonant with the relevant research findings. No study, including our own, which reports on the childhood experiences of an extremely impaired group of inpatients, has found that all borderline patients report having been sexually abused, and not all sexually abused patients in these studies are borderline. Rather, the majority of studies have found that between 40% and 71% of borderline patients and between 19% and 26% of control subjects report some type of sexual abuse during childhood and/or adolescence. In addition, about 25% of borderline patients and 6%–12% of control subjects report some type of parent-child incest. The latter figure is particularly salient, because parent-child incest has been found to have more serious long-term consequences than any other type of sexual abuse (Browne and Finkelhor 1986; Herman et al. 1986). Additionally, the majority of abuse survivors do not seem to develop any type of serious adult psychopathology (Browne and Finkelhor 1986; Herman et al. 1986).

The most deleterious consequence of this belief in the etiological centrality of a childhood history of sexual abuse is that it seriously distorts the basic nature of psychotherapy and in so doing, robs it of much of its efficacy. At its best, psychotherapy consists of the construction of a life narrative that is true to the facts at hand and that leads to better functioning and a stable sense of self-esteem. Traditionally, the following three factors are present: 1) the patient takes the main role in the construction of this narrative, 2) both patient and therapist try to keep an open mind about its eventual nature and content, and 3) both patient and therapist try to make this narrative as complete as possible. Although those who believe that sexual abuse is the main etiological factor in the development of BPD are well intended, their approach inadvertently plays on areas of particular vulnerability for borderline patients. More specifically, borderline patients are in tremendous emotional pain and are eager to understand the factors that led to this pain. Borderline patients also long for a close, emotionally intense, even exclusive relationship with their therapist. The combination of a therapist who is sure of what went wrong in the patient's life and who is offering a simple (albeit emotionally charged) solution to a complex problem and a patient who is in enormous pain and who is longing for attention and closeness often leads to one of a number of negative outcomes. Five of these outcomes seem most salient.

First, borderline patients who have not been sexually abused are made to feel that their painful life experiences, which may have included years of emotional torture and an almost complete denial of their feelings and thoughts, are trivial and even irrelevant. The life experiences of borderline patients who have not been severely sexually abused may also be trivialized. Plainly, the contemplative work of psychotherapy is much more difficult in an environment where pain has become a competitive sport.

Second, patients may become so desperate to please their therapist and so confused about the actual facts of their life that they may exaggerate the extent of their abuse history or even fabricate one. Although these situations are rare, they are tragic for the individual patient in that the source of his or her pain is still unknown and yet to be addressed. Such situations are also tragic for the borderline patients who have accurately reported the details of their history of sexual abuse, because they fuel the existing skepticism about the veracity of their accounts.

Third, patients may become so dependent on their therapist and so enmeshed with him or her that they dutifully continue to uncover and relive abuse memories even though their basic functioning is deteriorating and their self-destructiveness is increasing. This unfortunate pattern has been well described by Herman (1992), who recommends that abuse issues be dealt with only after the patients' impulsivity has decreased and their ability to care for themselves has stabilized.

Fourth, patients may end up taking a passive role in the construction of their life narrative, never determining what they think has been most traumatic in their life. Although sexual abuse may be the childhood event most horrific to the clinician, our clinical experience suggests that it may not be so to all patients. Rather, it may be emblematic of the ongoing chaos and insensitivity that they faced daily—a chaos and insensitivity that left them with chronic feelings of helplessness, worthlessness, and inchoate rage.

Fifth, patients may never explore the complexity of their history. Instead of remembering and reliving the full array of their painful life experiences, they may continue to ignore, deny, or belittle the other ways they have been abused, the ways they have been neglected, the effect of early separations on their abandonment fears, and the enormous strain of living with an emotionally ill caretaker.

LIMITATIONS OF THE PRESENT STUDY AND DIRECTIONS FOR FUTURE RESEARCH

The major limitation of the present study is that data relevant to all the important parameters of childhood sexual abuse were not systematically collected for all patients: age at onset, duration, frequency, relationship to perpetrator, use of force, and type of sexual activity. Another limitation of the present study is that its findings may not be generalizable to less severely disturbed outpatients.

In terms of future research, studies of carefully defined cohorts of borderline patients are needed that simultaneously investigate basic temperament, a full range of pathological and protective childhood experiences, caretaker psychopathology to which patients may have been exposed, and the possible genetic influence of a family history of selected psychiatric disorders. Longitudinal studies are also needed that prospectively assess the effects of childhood sexual abuse on the adult functioning of borderline patients. In addition, studies of children at high risk for developing BPD are needed. We are currently engaged in such a multidimensional study and hope that the results will expand our knowledge concerning both the etiology and course of BPD.

CONCLUSIONS

The most striking characteristics of borderline patients are the enormity of their inner pain and their understandable demand that we pay attention to this pain (Zanarini and Frankenburg 1994). We now know that many of their complaints are fully justified. They have typically been deeply hurt in childhood and need our validation of these painful experiences to begin and sustain their journey to health.

Overall, the results of this study suggest that childhood sexual abuse is neither necessary nor sufficient for the development of BPD. For about half of our borderline patients, childhood sexual abuse appears to be an important etiological factor. However, this abuse usually seems to be embedded in an atmosphere of general chaos and biparental neglect. For the other half of our patients, other forms of abuse (i.e., emotional abuse, verbal abuse, and physical abuse), in conjunction with various forms of neglect, probably play a more central etiological role.

In time, we will understand the etiology of BPD more fully. Although enormous strides have been made in the last decade, research into the multifactorial basis of BPD is still in its infancy. For now, we suggest that one can admire borderline patients for the integrity with which they have dealt with their pain. After all, not many people remain so loyal to and so respectful of such disheartening childhood experiences.

REFERENCES

Akiskal HS, Chen SE, Davis GC, et al: Borderline: an adjective in search of a noun. J Clin Psychiatry 46:41–48, 1985

Bradley SJ: The relationship of early maternal separation to borderline personality in children and adolescents: a pilot study. Am J Psychiatry 136:424–426, 1979

Browne A, Finkelhor D: Impact of child sexual abuse: a review of the research. Psychol Bull 99:66–77, 1986

Clarkin JF, Hull JW, Cantor J, et al: Borderline personality disorder and personality traits: a comparison of SCID-II BPD and NEO-PI. Psychological Assessment 5:472–476, 1993

Coccaro EF, Siever LJ, Klar HM, et al: Serotonergic studies in patients with affective and personality disorders: correlates with suicidal and impulsive aggressive behavior. Arch Gen Psychiatry 46:587–599, 1989

Frank H, Hoffman N: Borderline empathy: an empirical investigation. Compr Psychiatry 27:387–395, 1986

Frank H, Paris J: Recollections of family experience in borderline patients. Arch Gen Psychiatry 38:1031–1034, 1981

Goldberg RL, Mann LS, Wise TN, et al: Parental qualities as perceived by borderline personality disorders. Hillside Journal of Clinical Psychiatry 7:134–140, 1985

Grinker RR, Werble B, Drye RC: The Borderline Syndrome: A Behavioral Study of Ego-Functions. New York, Basic Books, 1968

Gunderson J, Kerr J, Englund D: The families of borderlines: a comparative study. Arch Gen Psychiatry 37:27–33, 1980

Herman JL: Trauma and Recovery. New York, Basic Books, 1992

Herman JL, van der Kolk BA: Traumatic antecedents of borderline personality disorder, in Psychological Trauma. Edited by van der Kolk BA. Washington, DC, American Psychiatric Press, 1987, pp 111–126

Herman J, Russell D, Trocki K: Long-term effects of incestuous abuse in childhood. Am J Psychiatry 143:1293–1296, 1986

Herman JL, Perry JC, van der Kolk BA: Childhood trauma in borderline personality disorder. Am J Psychiatry 146:490–495, 1989

Links PS, Steiner M, Offord DR, et al: Characteristics of borderline personality disorder: a Canadian study. Can J Psychiatry 33:336–340, 1988

Ogata SN, Silk KR, Goodrich S, et al: Childhood sexual and physical abuse in adult patients with borderline personality disorder. Am J Psychiatry 147:1008–1013, 1990

Paris J, Frank H: Perceptions of parental bonding in borderline patients. Am J Psychiatry 146:1498–1499, 1989

Salzman JP, Salzman C, Wolfson AN, et al: Association between borderline personality structure and history of childhood abuse in adult volunteers. Compr Psychiatry 34:254–257, 1993

Shearer SL, Peters CP, Quaytman MS, et al: Frequency and correlates of childhood sexual and physical abuse histories in adult female borderline inpatients. Am J Psychiatry 147:214–216, 1990

Soldz S, Budman S, Demby A, et al: Representation of personality disorders in circumplex and five-factor space: explorations with a clinical sample. Psychological Assessment 5:41–52, 1993

Soloff PH, Millward JW: Developmental histories of borderline patients. Compr Psychiatry 24:574–588, 1983

Spitzer RL, Williams JBW, Gibbon M, et al: Structured Clinical Interview for DSM-III-R Axis I Disorders. Washington, DC, American Psychiatric Press, 1990

Trull TJ: DSM-III-R personality disorders and the five-factor model of personality: an empirical comparison. J Abnorm Psychol 101:553–560, 1992

Walsh F: The family of the borderline patient, in The Borderline Patient. Edited by Grinker RR, Werble B. New York, Jason Aronson, 1977, pp 158–177

Westen D, Ludolph P, Misle B, et al: Physical and sexual abuse in adolescent girls with borderline personality disorder. Am J Orthopsychiatry 60:55–66, 1990

Zanarini MC, Frankenburg FR: Emotional hypochondriasis, hyperbole, and the borderline patient. Journal of Psychotherapy Practice and Research 3:25–36, 1994

Zanarini MC, Weinberg E: Borderline personality disorder: impulsive and compulsive features, in Impulsivity and Compulsivity. Edited by Oldham JM, Hollander E, Skodol AE. Washington, DC, American Psychiatric Press, 1996, pp 37–58

Zanarini MC, Frankenburg FR, Chauncey DL, et al: The Diagnostic Interview for Personality Disorders: interrater and test-retest reliability. Compr Psychiatry 28:467–480, 1987

Zanarini MC, Gunderson JG, Marino MF, et al: Childhood experiences of borderline patients. Compr Psychiatry 30:18–25, 1989a

Zanarini MC, Gunderson JG, Frankenburg FR, et al: The Revised Diagnostic Interview for Borderlines: discriminating BPD from other Axis II disorders. Journal of Personality Disorders 3:10–18, 1989b

Zanarini MC, Kimble CR, Williams AA: Neurological dysfunction in borderline patients and Axis II control subjects, in Biological and Neurobehavioral Studies of Borderline Personality Disorder. Edited by Silk KR. Washington, DC, American Psychiatric Press, 1994, pp 159–175

Chapter 4

Etiological Factors in a Sample of Convicted Women Felons in North Carolina

B. Kathleen Jordan, Ph.D., William E. Schlenger, Ph.D., Juesta M. Caddell, Ph.D., and John A. Fairbank, Ph.D.

Although perspectives on biological and environmental factors that may influence the development of borderline personality disorder (BPD) have evolved over time, for the past few decades there has been a consensus among researchers and clinicians that relationships with significant others while growing up (particularly caretakers) play a key role in the development of the disorder. Childhood experiences reported in the literature as being associated with BPD include

- Loss of or separation from a parent (Links et al. 1988; Paris et al. 1988; Snyder et al. 1985)
- Neglect, parental overprotectiveness, and "affectless control" by one or both parents (Paris and Frank 1989; Westen et al. 1990; Zanarini et al. 1989a; Zweig-Frank and Paris 1991)
- Sexual and/or physical abuse (Goldman et al. 1992; Goodwin et al. 1990; Herman et al. 1989; Links et al. 1988; Lobel 1992; Ogata et al. 1990; Westen et al. 1990; Zanarini et al. 1989a)
- Other problems with parents and in the family, such as having a parent with a psychiatric disorder (Paris et al. 1988; Schulz et al. 1989; Snyder et al. 1985; Zanarini et al. 1989a)

However, none of these factors has been found to be universally related to BPD, and some may be associated with subgroups of those with BPD. For example, in some studies, it appears that having been the victim of abuse is associated with having more severe symptoms of BPD (Salzman et al. 1993; Stone et al. 1988; Westen et al. 1990).

Researchers have also examined whether sociodemographic characteristics, such as gender, race and ethnicity, and age, may be related to BPD. Sociodemographic characteristics reported in the literature as being associated with elevated rates of BPD include gender (female), age (younger), and urbanicity (more urban). Results for racial and ethnic status have been mixed. Generally, race and ethnicity have not been found to be related to having a diagnosis of BPD. In some studies, however, the prevalence of BPD has been reported to be elevated for one or more racial and ethnic groups, although the racial and ethnic groups reported as having elevated rates vary across studies (Akhtar et al. 1986; Castaneda and Franco 1985; Snyder et al. 1985; Swartz et al. 1990).

Many of the results described above come from studies of patient samples. However, examining the sociodemographic characteristics, level of symptomatology, and other correlates of a specific psychiatric disorder in nonpatient samples may provide a more comprehensive portrait of a disorder than can be seen by examining exclusively individuals who seek treatment. This group may differ in important ways (e.g., level of symptomatology, socioeconomic status) from individuals with the disorder who do not seek treatment. It may be that symptom profiles, co-occurring disorders, and etiological factors for individuals in nontreatment populations are different from those for individuals in treatment populations.

Ideally, one would like to examine the disorder and its correlates by using as research subjects random samples of individuals in the community who have BPD (regardless of their treatment status). However, it would be 1) expensive and time consuming to screen large numbers of community residents for the disorder to find subjects and 2) difficult to obtain large samples of such individuals.

One approach for studying a disorder in nonpatient samples is to use as subjects individuals from nonpatient groups in which one might expect to find an elevated rate of the disorder of interest. (Although these are also "special samples," and findings from such studies are also not generalizable to untreated individuals in the general community, the approach nonetheless gives the researcher an opportunity to examine the robustness of the findings from treatment samples.) Because individuals with BPD often exhibit behaviors (e.g., illicit drug use and reckless driving) that can bring them to the attention of criminal-justice authorities, one might expect to find an elevated prevalence of BPD among women criminal offenders. It is also a group in which those with BPD may differ in important ways from women in treatment-seeking samples, such as racial and/or ethnic characteristics and socioeconomic status.

A recent study of women prison inmates in North Carolina provides the opportunity to examine the ways in which women with BPD in prison might differ from women in treatment-seeking samples and thus to increase the understanding of the phenomenology and correlates of the disorder across a broad spectrum of individuals with the disorder. The sample used in this study of women inmates, for example, had a majority of nonwhite women, a group that has been underrepresented in studies of BPD. Learning more about BPD among women inmates has another potential benefit as well. Because many symptoms of BPD, such as impulsiveness and involvement with drugs, are behaviors that can lead to arrest and rearrest, a better understanding of BPD among convicted women felons can inform policies regarding psychiatric treatment of women in prison, and prevention/recidivism programs for women currently in prison or at risk of being sent to prison.

In this chapter we examine risk factors for BPD, using data collected from an in-depth survey and structured clinical interviews with women prison inmates in North Carolina, all of whom had been convicted of a felony. We first provide distributions on a set of sociodemographic, etiological, and other variables (e.g., personal and lifestyle characteristics, including comparisons of those with and without BPD). Then we present results from a multivariate analysis of potential risk factors for BPD. These results allow examination of the relative importance of multiple risk factors in this population while controlling for other such factors. Finally, we discuss some implications of these findings.

STUDY DESIGN

The data in this chapter come from the Women Inmates' Health Study (WIHS), the most comprehensive study conducted so far in the United States of the psychosocial status of women prison inmates (Jordan et al. 1992). The WIHS differed from most previous studies of women inmates in several important ways. First, to avoid the bias associated with special samples of women criminal offenders (e.g., those sent for forensic evaluation), we included a virtual census of inmates who entered prison during the period of the study. Second, we conducted interviews with more subjects than were interviewed in most previous studies ($N = 805$). The large sample size allowed for more stable prevalence estimates than in most previous studies. Third, the administration of a 2½-hour structured survey interview allowed us to assess more covariates than have been examined in many previous studies.

Between July 1991 and November 1992, all women felons newly sentenced to prison in North Carolina were asked to participate in the study, which used a two-stage design that is common in community epidemiological studies (Dohrenwend and Shrout 1981). The first stage was a survey interview with all subjects in the sample ($N = 805$). The in-depth, face-to-face survey interviews were conducted in private by a professional survey interviewer trained in the administration of the instrument. The interviewer explained that participation was voluntary and that all information was confidential. The response rate was 95%.

The second stage of the study was a follow-up interview with about one-quarter (210) of the respondents who had been interviewed in the survey component of the study. This follow-up interview was included to validate the diagnosis of BPD and posttraumatic stress disorder (PTSD) that was developed with the survey instrumentation. In the follow-up component, trained clinicians administered the PTSD module of the Structured Clinical Interview for DSM-III-R (SCID; Spitzer et al. 1987) and the Revised Diagnostic Interview for Borderlines (DIB-R; Zanarini et al. 1989b). The response rate for the clinical substudy was 98%.

Assessment of Psychiatric Disorder

Three disorders key to the analyses described here are BPD, PTSD, and antisocial personality disorder (ASPD). For the WIHS, we used the DSM-III-R (American Psychiatric Association 1987) definitions for BPD, PTSD, and ASPD.

According to DSM-III-R, to be categorized as having PTSD, one must have experienced one or more extreme events—events that are "outside the range of usual human experience" and that "would be markedly distressing to almost anyone" (American Psychiatric Association 1987, p. 247). These include, but are not limited to, such events as rape, incest, physical assault, fires, serious accidents, and natural disasters. In addition to exposure to an extreme event, the person must present with other symptoms, including 1) persistent reexperiencing of the event, 2) numbing of responsiveness to or persistent avoidance of people, places, things, or thoughts associated with the trauma, and 3) persistent symptoms of arousal not present before the trauma.

ASPD is characterized as a pattern of irresponsible and antisocial behavior beginning in childhood or early adolescence and continuing into adulthood.

In the main survey sample, BPD was assessed with a modification of the BPD module of the Revised Diagnostic Interview for Personality Disorders (DIPD-R; Zanarini et al. 1987). This module uses DSM-III-R criteria for BPD and has been found to have satisfactory reliability. The instrument was adapted for use in the WIHS to 1) allow for administration by an interviewer who was not a clinician but a trained lay survey interviewer and 2) ensure that women with low levels of education and little or no experience or knowledge of psychological constructs would be able to understand and answer the questions. With the DSM-III-R diagnosis of BPD from the DIB-R as the referent for validation, the survey measure of BPD correctly classified 167 of the 210 clinical sample subjects (79%) and had a sensitivity of 77% and a specificity of 81%.

ASPD was assessed with a module from the Diagnostic Interview Schedule (DIS; Robins et al. 1981). The DIS is a structured interview developed for administration by lay interviewers. It has a number of modules, each assessing a different psychiatric disorder. The DIS has demonstrated acceptable reliability and validity for most disorders (Robins et al. 1981, 1982).

Because there is no interview schedule to assess PTSD that 1) has been designed for administration by professional survey interviewers and 2) has been validated on samples of subjects who were not in treatment, we included the Impact of Events Scale (IES; Horwitz et al. 1979) to assess PTSD. We used a version of the IES that had been expanded in a previous study to include items assessing the B, C, and D criteria for PTSD shown in DSM-III-R (Weiss 1993). We hoped that using the IES diagnostically would allow us to develop a measure of PTSD "caseness" that was concordant with a clinical PTSD diagnosis as determined in our follow-up clinical interviews that used the SCID's PTSD module.

It should be noted that several other disorders (although not the focus of this chapter) were assessed in this study, including major depression, dysthymia, panic disorder, generalized anxiety disorder, and substance abuse.

Assessment of Trauma

One important component of the study was the assessment of exposure to psychological trauma. Anecdotal and preliminary research evidence suggested that exposure to extreme (psychologically traumatic) events was common in this population, and we thought important treatment and policy implications might be found in an examination of the prevalence, nature, and outcomes of such exposure. In the survey interview, we asked respondents a lengthy series of very explicit questions to determine whether they had experienced particular types of events. Specific questions were asked to detail women's experiences of a broad range of extreme events (e.g., sexual and physical assault, accidents, natural disasters). These questions were a modification and expansion of items used by Kilpatrick and colleagues at the Medical University of South Carolina to assess respondents' history of exposure to sexual assault (Falsetti et al. 1994). We did not assess inmates' experience of psychological or emotional abuse or neglect.

Potential Predispositional Factors Examined in the Multivariate Analyses of BPD

In these analyses, we examined the relationship of a group of potential risk factors and control variables to BPD in a multivariate framework, using logistic regression. In this case, the dependent variable was a current diagnosis of BPD. Logistic regression, because it is a multivariate technique, permits the researcher to examine simultaneously the relationship of multiple potential risk factors and control variables to BPD. Doing so allows the researcher to determine the individual contribution of each set of potential risk factors while controlling for both other risk factors and control variables. A number of variables, consisting of potential risk factors in the child's home life while she was growing up, were examined. Most of the independent or "predictor" variables available to us and included in the analyses have been previously examined in studies of risk factors for BPD (e.g., age, race, urbanicity, loss of or separation from a parent, and physical and sexual abuse). We also included other variables that we hypothesized might be related to BPD (e.g., the overall level of family violence and the number of conduct disorder symptom groups). Additionally, bed-wetting after age 6 was included because it was found by Robins (1966) to be predisposing for ASPD, and ASPD is one of the control variables used in the analysis. Overall, the following 15 predictor variables were studied: age, race, urbanicity, bed-wetting after age 6, family violence, economic and physical deprivation index, other family problems (e.g., psychiatric disorders and/or antisocial behavior), feeling safe and protected, loss, number of conduct disorder groups, sexual assault before age 11, physical assault before age 11, other traumatic event before age 11, ASPD, and PTSD.

As described in the opening of this chapter, many studies have reported that abuse or assault while growing up is associated with the development of BPD, although these findings differ in 1) whether it is physical or sexual abuse that is associated with BPD and 2) the proportion of those with BPD who have experienced such a victimization. Some previous studies do not clearly specify the age at which the abuse had to occur in order to be included as "abuse" in the analyses. Thus, differences in the age at which the abuse occurred may be a factor in differences in findings across studies. Personality disorders in general, and BPD specifically, are widely believed to have their roots in childhood, so we chose to focus on childhood experiences. Examining childhood traumatic experiences was also important because there is evidence that if abuse or assault occurs in childhood, it is more pathogenic and leads to poorer outcomes than if the experience occurs at a later age, such as in adolescence (Courtois 1979; Meiselman 1978; Paris and Zweig-Frank 1992). We therefore limited our examination to physical and sexual abuse (examined separately) that occurred in childhood (i.e., before the onset of adolescence). Because both the age at menarche and the age at which children begin to take on adolescent roles have declined in recent decades, we defined *childhood* as before age 11, and we included in our analysis only abuse that occurred before age 11. We also examined the effects of other types of trauma that occurred before age 11 (e.g., being in a serious natural disaster or observing severe violence).

Another reason for differences in findings across studies may be the lack of a clear and accepted definition of *abuse*. In our analysis, any one of the three types of childhood trauma (sexual abuse, physical abuse, other trauma) was required to meet the DSM-III-R definition of an extreme event, as described previously. In our coding of experiences, most sexual interactions between the respondent before age 11 and an adult were considered to meet DSM-III-R criteria for psychological trauma. For physical abuse, however, the beating or other assault had to be fairly severe to be considered "out of the range of normal human experience" (e.g., the assault resulted in bruising or necessitated that the respondent stay in bed for a day or more or see a doctor). If the experience was not serious enough to meet these criteria, physical abuse was coded as "absent."

One additional factor that may play a role in differences across studies is the other set of covariates included in the analyses. Our study gave us the opportunity to examine, simultaneously, the effects of physical and sexual abuse and other potential risk factors. One of the advantages of logistic regression is that one can control for factors that may obscure or confuse the findings. For example, age, gender, and race and ethnicity are often included as control variables in logistic regressions because the independent variables may affect the dependent variable differently, depending on the individual's age, gender, or race and ethnicity. In our analyses, PTSD and ASPD were included as control variables because of the high degree of co-occurrence of BPD with PTSD and ASPD in this sample. By including PTSD and ASPD as independent variables in the logistic regression, we were able to determine what the predisposing factors were for BPD, excluding the factors that were predisposing for the other co-occurring disorder.

To conduct the regression, we used a forward solution with backward elimination. Only the variables with a significance level of .05 were retained.

RESULTS

Demographics and Family Environment While Growing Up

The majority of WIHS inmates were nonwhite (64%; 515) (most of this group was black), were between the ages of 21 and 34 (68%; 547; mean age = 31), had less than 12 years of education (54%; 435), were mothers (77%; 620) of more than one child (53%; 427), and had less than $2,000 in personal income in the year before entrance to prison (67%; 539). At the time they entered prison, 41% (330) reported that they had never been married (the most commonly reported marital status), 19% (153) reported that they had been living as married, and the remainder reported being married, separated, and divorced in about equal numbers. In general, there were no important racial and ethnic differences in the sociodemographic characteristics of our sample.

There were family problems in many of these women's backgrounds. The majority of the women (60%; 483) did not live with both of their natural parents until age 16. While they were growing up, a substantial minority saw their parents hitting each other (34%; 274) and/or had a family or household member who had a problem with drug abuse (13%; 105) or alcohol abuse (41%; 330), had a serious mental health problem (20%; 161), or was involved with the criminal justice system (e.g., 28% [225] had a family member who had served time in jail or prison).

Criminal Status and History

Almost half of the sample (46%; 370) were in prison for the first time, and only 14.5% (117) had been in jail, prison, or a detention center before age 18. The majority of the women were in prison for drug use, possession, or sale; forgery; bad checks; and/or probation or parole violations. Only 11% (89) were in prison for any kind of violent assault. The most common offenses for which WIHS inmates had been arrested previously were the same as those for which they were currently incarcerated, with the addition of theft/larceny. It was also unusual for the inmates in our sample to have been arrested for violence previously—only 16% (129) had been arrested on a violent-assault charge previously.

Psychological Trauma

A large majority (78%; 628) had experienced a traumatic event that met DSM-III-R criteria for an "extreme event." Not surprisingly, physical and sexual assaults, including childhood physical and sexual abuse, were the most common types of extreme/traumatic events reported by respondents (61% [491] reported abuse or assaults). Many respondents had been exposed to more than one psychologically traumatic event as a child, as an adult, or both.

Prevalence of Specific Psychiatric Disorders

BPD, ASPD, and PTSD all appear to be more prevalent in this population than in the general community population. Approximately 28% (225) of the sample met DSM-III-R diagnostic criteria for (current) BPD, and approximately 11% (89) of the sample met criteria for (current) ASPD. For comparison, Epidemiologic Catchment Area (ECA) investigators, using data from community populations, have estimated the 1-year prevalence of BPD to be 1.8%—although the rate for women would be slightly higher (Swartz et al. 1990)—and the 1-month prevalence of ASPD for women to be 0.2% (Regier et al. 1988).

At this time, we are unable to provide a psychometrically sound estimate for the rate of PTSD for our study population. None of the algorithms we have used for scoring the survey interview PTSD module has had good concordance with the clinical PTSD diagnosis. Therefore, we have provided what we consider conservative and liberal estimates of the rate of PTSD in this population, labeled PTSD I and PTSD II, respectively (see Table 4–1). These rates represent two ways of scoring the IES, using the overall IES score and the total score for items assessing the C and D criteria. Our lifetime estimates are 30% (242) and 39% (314). The reported prevalence of PTSD in community samples ranges from 1% to 28% (Davidson and Fairbank 1993).

Comorbidity

The majority of those with BPD also either had ASPD or appeared to have PTSD. Of those with BPD, 26% (58) met criteria for ASPD; between 50% (111) and 61% (135) of those with BPD appeared to also have PTSD. About half of the sample appeared to have one or more of these disorders, and about 5% (36–42) appeared to have all three.

Descriptive Analysis of Differences in Characteristics and Behaviors

Tables 4–2 and 4–3 present descriptive findings for some key etiological variables as well as for some salient adult behaviors and characteristics. Table 4–2 provides comparisons between those without and with BPD by showing percentages of these groups that answered "yes" to questions on some salient dichotomous variables, such as whether the respondent lived with her natural mother and father until the age of 16. This table also includes the χ^2 value and associated probability for the differences in proportion between the two groups. Table 4–3 provides the means of some salient continuous variables for those without and with BPD. The results of t tests are also presented in this table.

Many of the women inmates in our sample were from troubled families, had had difficulties growing up, had had trouble with the law, and had had mental health, alcohol, and drug problems.

Table 4–1.   Number and percentage for diagnosis groups ($N = 805$)

Diagnosis	N	%
Using PTSD I		
BPD only	89	11.1
ASPD only	25	3.1
PTSD I only	121	15.0
BPD and ASPD	22	2.7
BPD and PTSD I	75	9.3
ASPD and PTSD I	7	0.9
BPD, ASPD, and PTSD I	36	4.5
None of these	428	53.1
Missing on diagnosis	2	0.2
Using PTSD II		
BPD only	71	8.8
ASPD only	23	2.9
PTSD II only	167	20.7
BPD and ASPD	16	2.0
BPD and PTSD II	93	11.5
ASPD and PTSD II	9	1.1
BPD, ASPD, and PTSD II	42	5.2
None of these	382	47.4
Missing on diagnosis	2	0.2

But even in this population, in which the base rate of problems is quite high, those with BPD tended to have more problems.

Fewer of those with BPD than those without BPD had lived with their natural parents until age 16 (Table 4–2). More of those with BPD had experienced a physical or sexual assault before age 11 or had experienced another type of psychological trauma by that age. More of those with BPD had also used illicit drugs, had used a needle to shoot up drugs in the past year, had received treatment for alcohol or drug problems, or had received inpatient or outpatient mental health care at some time in their lives. Finally, more of those with BPD had been arrested for a violent offense and/or had experienced a major depression in their lifetimes.

In Table 4–3, we see that those with BPD were slightly younger, had drunk more alcohol in the past year, had been arrested

Table 4–2. Percentage answering "yes" on dichotomous variables, for those without and those with borderline personality disorder (BPD)

	Without BPD	With BPD	χ^2	P
Lived with natural mother and father until age 16	44	30	12.3	> .001
Sexual assault before age 11	9	32	61.9	> .001
Physical assault before age 11	2	5	7.0	.008
Other trauma before age 11	5	10	5.8	.016
Has used illicit drugs	67	86	28.9	> .001
Has used a needle to shoot up drugs in the past year	15	26	10.3	.001
Has received treatment for alcohol or drug problems	35	64	56.7	> .001
Has received inpatient mental health care	9	29	51.7	> .001
Has received outpatient mental health care	11	40	86.7	> .001
Has been arrested for a violent offense at some time	14	23	10.1	.001
Has had a major depressive episode	5	32	104.8	> .001

much more often before age 15, and had had vaginal intercourse with more partners in the past year than had those without BPD. Women with BPD had also been arrested much more often since age 18. Although this difference did not reach statistical significance, it was probably due, at least in part, to the large variance for this variable.

Multivariate Analyses of BPD

PTSD II, the more "sensitive" of the two PTSD categorizations, was included as an independent variable in the regression analysis for control purposes. The decision to use PTSD II (rather than PTSD I) was based on the overarching rationale for including

Table 4–3. Mean differences in characteristics and behaviors between those without and those with borderline personality disorder (BPD)

Characteristic or behavior	Without BPD	With BPD	t	P
Age	31.4	29.3	3.8	> .001
Average number of alcoholic drinks had in 1 day in past year	6.6	11.0	−4.2	> .001
Number of times arrested before age 15	1.3	7.2	−3.1	.002
Number of men had vaginal intercourse with in past 12 months	3.2	6.2	−2.5	.012
Number of times arrested since age 18	6.4	12.3	−1.2	.230

PTSD in the analysis—that is, to prevent factors associated with PTSD from being mistakenly found to be explanatory for BPD. This more inclusive categorization of PTSD was used to ensure that all possible cases of PTSD were classified as positive for the disorder in the regression analyses.

Findings from the logistic regression are shown in Table 4–4. Family violence, other family problems, and sexual assault before age 11 were statistically significant predictors of BPD, as was a diagnosis of ASPD or PTSD. These latter variables also had the largest standardized coefficients and/or odds ratios. Having been sexually assaulted, having ASPD or PTSD, or having a violent family all approximately doubled the odds of having BPD. Although the odds ratio for family problem is smaller than those for the variables just mentioned, in fact, family problems appears to have a much more powerful effect, because this variable is not dichotomous but has a 6-point range. Therefore, the odds of developing BPD would increase substantially for individuals whose families exhibited several of the problems assessed.

The small odds ratio for age may also be misleading. Because age is a continuous variable with a range of approximately

Table 4–4. Logistic regression results, significant parameters only
(*N* = 805; dependent variable, BPD)

PP Variable	Standardized estimate	Adjusted odds ratio	*P*
ASPD	0.23	1.87	.0001
PTSD II	0.22	2.21	.0001
Family violence	0.18	1.88	.0013
Other family problems	0.19	1.26	.0003
Bed-wetting	−0.11	0.58	.0262
Sexual assault before age 11	0.15	2.02	.0016
Age	−0.11	0.98	.0442

Notes. Model χ^2 = 185, df = 7, and *P* of χ^2 = .0001; model R^2 = .17.
ASPD = antisocial personality disorder; BPD = borderline personality disorder;
PTSD = posttraumatic stress disorder.

18 to 70, in fact, the effect of age is also substantial for large age differences. for example, the odds of a woman inmate's having BPD at age 28 is .781 compared to women inmates of age 18.

Finally, bed-wetting was negatively associated with BPD (i.e., bed-wetting after age 6 was associated with not having BPD as an adult).

Variables that were not found to be significant predictors for BPD are also worth examining. Physical assault or other trauma before age 11 and loss of or separation from a parent, for example, were not significant predictors. Age, race, urbanicity, deprivation, and feeling in danger while growing up were also not significant predictors. Moreover, having a diagnosis of ASPD was not a significant predictor.

DISCUSSION

Multivariate Analysis

Variables Found to Be Predictive in the Regression Model

Our analyses were supportive of some previous research findings but also suggested some new relationships. Many previous studies have reported rates of childhood sexual abuse to be elevated among patients with BPD, compared either with (most often) other patients or with other control subjects (Herman et al. 1989; Links et al. 1988; Ogata et al. 1990; Westen et al. 1990; Zanarini et al. 1989a). Consistent with the literature, we found that even in a population in which early sexual assaults appear to be more common than in the general community population, and even in the context of a multivariate analysis that partials out the effects of other predispositional variables, sexual assault before age 11 is highly predictive of BPD.

Some previous studies have found no significant differences in the prevalence of childhood physical abuse in those with BPD as compared with others (Herman et al. 1989; Ogata et al. 1990; Westen et al. 1990; Zanarini et al. 1989a), whereas other studies have found such differences (Links et al. 1988). In our examination of the WIHS data, we found that although there was a statistically significant bivariate relationship between serious physical assault before age 11 and BPD, such an assault was not a significant predictor of BPD when other variables were controlled in the multivariate analyses. However, the overall level of violence in the family, examined less often in the etiological literature on BPD, was an important predictor. It appears that the women inmates with BPD tended to grow up in homes in which violence against at least some family members was common. The descriptive data, however, tell us that few of the women, either with or without BPD, reported being severely physically abused before age 11. Because the family violence variable included violence against the respondent that was less serious than experiencing a serious physical assault before age 11, and because family violence was reported much more frequently than were serious physical assaults against the respondent, the presence of the family violence variable in the multivariate analysis may have suppressed the bivariate relationship between serious physical assault before age 11 and BPD.

As cited in the introduction to this chapter, other family problems (i.e., those other than family violence) have also been reported to be elevated among those with BPD. The significance of the predictor "other family problems" in our regression analysis is consistent with this finding and reflects the troubled homes from which these women came. It appears that in addition to experiencing sexual assault, women with BPD who were in prison grew up in homes in which adult household and family members were likely to have problems not only with violent behavior but also with drugs, alcohol, criminal activities, and/or mental disorders. Furthermore, women inmates with BPD reported having come from family environments in which the level of family problems was sufficiently serious to distinguish these women's families from the families of other women in prison, many of whom also came from troubled home environments.

Another finding of note is that PTSD was a statistically significant predictor of BPD. Its contribution to the model was consistent with the comorbidity of BPD and PTSD in our sample. Some 50% or more of those with BPD also appeared to meet criteria for PTSD. Several investigators believe that BPD may be a complex, chronic variant of PTSD (Herman and van der Kolk 1987; Herman et al. 1986). The findings from this study offer support for the view that childhood trauma and its sequelae may be important factors in the development of both PTSD and BPD.

A high degree of comorbidity has been found among personality disorders in many studies. And, because there is overlap between behaviors associated with ASPD and behaviors associated with BPD (e.g., substance abuse), it is logical that, statistically, BPD would be related to ASPD. What is striking, however, is that this association holds up in a sample of women criminal offenders, because we would expect that many women in prison who did not have BPD would also exhibit elevated rates of antisocial symptoms.

It appears, however, that the women prison inmates in our sample generally did not exhibit the high level of antisocial behavior, as a child or as an adult, that is usually found among male prison inmates. In other analyses not described here, we found that about three-quarters of the women in our sample exhibited relatively low levels of violent behavior. This is consistent with the types of offenses for which these women have been incarcerated (e.g., drugs, forgery, bad checks). Only 15% of the sample met criteria for conduct disorder (that is, exhibited behaviors in three or more conduct disorder groups before age 15), and only 11% met criteria for ASPD. Therefore, the finding that ASPD is predictive of BPD in this sample does not appear to reflect an extremely high rate of ASPD among the women with BPD. (Only about one-quarter of those with BPD in this sample also met criteria for ASPD.) Rather, the association between ASPD and BPD appears to reflect the relatively low rate of ASPD, overall, among the women *without* BPD. Therefore, one cannot conclude from these data that the women with BPD in our sample have shown significantly more, or more serious, antisocial behaviors than have other women with BPD.

Nonetheless, the descriptive findings show that women inmates with BPD were more likely than other women inmates to report having been arrested for a violent offense and that they also reported more arrests before age 15 than did inmates without BPD. Together, these findings would tend to support the hypothesis that these women acted out from an early age. Further, one reason that these women with BPD have been incarcerated, when many other women with BPD have not been, may be that these women exhibited more, or more serious, troublesome behaviors than did other women with BPD.

Finally, as has been found in other studies of acting-out personality disorders, it appears that the rates of BPD decrease with age. In studies of those with ASPD, such declining rates have been attributed both to higher rates of acting-out behaviors of later cohorts and to the decreased acting out of individuals when they reach middle age (Robins 1989). Both of these factors may contribute to declining rates of BPD as well.

Variables Not Found to Be Predictive in the Regression Model

Race, deprivation, urbanicity, loss of or separation from a parent, and feeling endangered while growing up were not significant predictors of BPD in the logistic regression. Many of these variables have been found in some previous studies to be associated with BPD. Their lack of significant association with BPD in our regression analysis may be, at least in part, a result of examining these relationships in a multivariate rather than in a bivariate context. We comment, however, on other possible reasons why specific variables were not found to be significant predictors of BPD.

One variable that might have been hypothesized to be a significant predictor because of the findings of some previous studies is loss of or separation from a parent (Links et al. 1988; Paris et al. 1988; Snyder et al. 1985). We did find that those with BPD were less likely than others to have lived with their natural parents until age 16. It appears, however, that loss of or separation from a parent was not important enough in itself to add predictive power to the model. In part, it may not be the loss per se so much as the conditions likely to occur with loss (e.g., "family problems") that are most predisposing to BPD. As for lack of significance of "feeling endangered," it is likely that the variables "sexual assaults before age 11" and "other family problems" are associated with feelings of danger, so that feeling endangered does not add much incrementally to the predictive power of the model.

We have hypotheses about the lack of significance of some other variables in the model as well. Physical neglect, which was not significant in our model, has not been found consistently to be a predictor of BPD, so our finding is consistent with at least some previous research. In addition, the sample tended to be somewhat homogeneous with respect to financial resources, and two of the three items in the index that assessed neglect were measures of poverty and financial need.

The lack of differences by urbanicity is not surprising because of the geographic location from which the sample was drawn. These women all were arrested and tried in North Carolina, and most are from North Carolina. This state has little in the way of true inner-city environments such as those in the larger metropolitan areas of New York City or Chicago. It is likely that the chaos and extreme harshness of family life in inner cities are an important source of differences between more- and less-urban groups in other studies.

Fit of the Model

In addition to examining the statistically significant predictors in the logistic regression model, it is important to examine the overall fit of the model. The model for BPD is statistically significant ($\chi^2 = 162$, $P < .0001$) and accounts for the equivalent of about 17% of the variance (pseudo R^2; Aldrich and Nelson 1984) in the

BPD diagnosis. Together, these two pieces of information suggest that the variables in the model reflect important risk factors for the development of BPD but that the model is underspecified. That is, other factors not included in this model account for 83% of the variance. These other factors may include vulnerabilities not measured in this study (e.g., biological predisposition) and/or other aspects of the family dynamics or experiences growing up. Nonetheless, the variance accounted for by variables in the model (17%) does represent an important advance in understanding the risk for developing BPD and is similar to the level of variance typically explained in such models.

Other Descriptive Findings

We also mention some other findings, unrelated to predispositional factors, that can help us to understand better how women in prison with BPD are similar to or different from other women with BPD. Consistent with the literature, in our analysis of the WIHS data, we found that depression was much more common among those with BPD than those without: one-third of those with BPD met criteria for a major depressive episode. Overall, the rate of depression was not elevated in the inmate sample as compared with community samples in North Carolina. Another interesting finding is that many of those with BPD had received treatment at some point in their lives: 29% inpatient mental health, 40% outpatient mental health, and 64% drug or alcohol. Therefore, there appears to be some overlap between this sample and treatment-seeking samples, particularly in public hospitals and clinics. Another notable result was that a greater proportion of those with BPD than without it had used illicit drugs (in a sample in which the majority had used drugs), and a greater proportion had also used a needle for drug use in the year before entering prison. This finding has important implications for the prevention of the spread of HIV (the human immunodeficiency virus).

Strengths and Limitations of the Study

The findings described in this chapter are based on self-reports and as such are subject to recall bias and intentional misrepresentation. However, there was no incentive for the women to overreport abuse or other problems and no disincentive for reporting their own troublesome behaviors. Interviewers reported that participants appeared to be quite frank, often becoming observably emotional in discussing distressing experiences. We believe that for most inmates, the responses they gave us were as accurate as they were able to provide.

One strength of our study is the size of our sample. It is unlikely that variables were found not to be significant because of lack of statistical power. Another strength is the large numbers included in our sample of 1) minorities, 2) individuals from the lower social strata, and 3) individuals who have never been treated for a psychiatric disorder. These factors provide us with information that allows us to understand better the precursors of BPD in individuals who have been understudied previously.

SUMMARY

As seen in the logistic regression results, our findings suggest that the etiological factors associated with BPD among women prisoners are similar to those found for women with BPD in other samples—childhood sexual abuse and a variety of problems with their parent(s) and in the family. Additionally, the significance of the family violence variable suggests that violence was likely to be present in the homes of many women with BPD while they were growing up, even though any physical abuse of the respondent before age 11 rarely met our severity criteria. The significance of the PTSD variable is consistent with the strong relationship that has often been found between early trauma, PTSD, and BPD. Finally, an ASPD diagnosis was found to be significantly related to BPD.

Summarizing some the important findings from the descriptive analyses, we found that women inmates with BPD were similar to women with BPD in other samples with respect to the co-occurrence of depression, involvement with one or more types of treatment, and abuse of drugs and alcohol. Further research is needed, however, to examine how the levels of several types of problems (such as the number of conduct disorder symptom groups, the extent of substance abuse, and the number of treatment episodes) are similar to, or different from, the levels in women with BPD in other samples.

IMPLICATIONS FOR CONCEPTUAL MODELS

The findings from our multivariate analyses provide evidence in support of conceptual models that assert that the development of borderline psychopathology "arises out of a history in which abusive experiences join other factors to help shape enduring aspects of the character" (Gunderson and Sabo 1993, p. 23). Among the factors that theorists have hypothesized as being related to the development of BPD are a variety of problems with primary caretakers, and our findings would tend to support these theories. Family problems, which is an index of several such problems, and family violence were both significant predictors of BPD in our multivariate analysis. Another predispositional factor predicated in some models is the loss of or separation from a parent. Consistent with this, the between-group relationship of parental loss or separation was also statistically significant. The fact that this relationship did not hold up in the multivariate analysis suggests that parental loss or separation may "operate through" other family problems in the development of BPD. That is, family problems may mediate the effect of parental loss or separation. Only recently have theorists come to incorporate the role of actual physical and/or sexual abuse in the development of the disorder. As the quotation from Gunderson and Sabo suggests, abusive experiences are now considered by many theorists to be important predispositional factors, at least for some individuals. Support for this theory also can be found in our regression analysis. Both our childhood sexual abuse variable and our PTSD variable were found to be significant predictors of BPD in this model.

OTHER IMPLICATIONS

Finally, it is important to note that alarmingly high numbers of women, nearly half of the entire sample, have serious problems associated with BPD and/or PTSD, and the majority of the sample members reported a history of psychological trauma. These findings suggest a need for treatment of sequelae to trauma for women in prison. Such treatment could help not only to alleviate the symptoms of these disorders but also to reduce recidivism, HIV risk, and transmission of problems to the children of these troubled women.

REFERENCES

Akhtar S, Byrne JP, Doghramji K: The demographic profile of borderline personality disorder. J Clin Psychiatry 47:196–198, 1986

Aldrich JH, Nelson FD: Linear Probability, Logit and Probit Models. London, Sage, 1984

American Psychiatric Association: Diagnostic and Statistical Manual of Mental Disorders, 3rd Edition, Revised. Washington, DC, American Psychiatric Association, 1987

Castaneda R, Franco H: Sex and ethnic distribution of borderline personality disorder in an inpatient sample. Am J Psychiatry 142:1202–1203, 1985

Courtois C: The incest experience and its aftermath. Victimology: An International Journal 4:337–347, 1979

Davidson JRT, Fairbank JA: The epidemiology of posttraumatic stress disorder, in Posttraumatic Stress Disorder: DSM-IV and Beyond. Edited by Davidson JRT, Foa EB. Washington, DC, American Psychiatric Press, 1993, pp 147–169

Dohrenwend B, Shrout P: Toward the development of a two-stage procedure for case identification and classification in psychiatric epidemiology. Research in Community and Mental Health 2:295–323, 1981

Falsetti SA, Resnick MS, Kilpatrick DG, et al: a review of the "Potential Stressful Events Interview": a comparative assessment instrument of high and low magnitude stressors. Behavior Therapist 17:66–67, 1994

Goldman SJ, D'Angelo EJ, DeMaso DR, et al: Physical and sexual abuse among children with borderline personality disorder. Am J Psychiatry 149:1723–1726, 1992

Goodwin JM, Cheeves K, Connell V: Borderline and other severe symptoms in adult survivors of incestuous abuse. Psychiatric Annals 20:22–32, 1990

Gunderson JG, Sabo AN: The phenomenological and conceptual interface between borderline personality disorder and PTSD. Am J Psychiatry 150:19–27, 1993

Herman JL, van der Kolk BA: Traumatic antecedents of BPD, in Psychological Trauma. Edited by van der Kolk BA. Washington, DC, American Psychiatric Press, 1987, pp 111–126

Herman J, Russel D, Trocki K: Long term effects of incestuous abuse in childhood. Am J Psychiatry 143:1293–1296, 1986

Herman JL, Perry JC, van der Kolk BA: Childhood trauma in borderline personality disorder. Am J Psychiatry 146:490–495, 1989

Horwitz M, Wilner N, Alvarez W: Impact of Events Scale: a measure of subject stress. Psychosom Med 41:209–218, 1979

Jordan BK, Schlenger WE, Fairbank JA, et al: The Women Inmates' Health Study: an overview. Paper presented at the annual meeting of the American Public Health Association, Washington, DC, November 1992

Links PS, Steiner M, Offord DR, et al: Characteristics of borderline personality disorder: a Canadian study. Can J Psychiatry 33:336–340, 1988

Lobel CM: Relationship between childhood sexual abuse and borderline personality disorder in women psychiatric inpatients. Journal of Child Sexual Abuse 1:63–80, 1992

Meiselman K: Incest. San Francisco, CA, Jossey-Bass, 1978

Ogata SN, Silk KR, Goodrich S, et al: Childhood sexual and physical abuse in adult patients with borderline personality disorder. Am J Psychiatry 147:1008–1013, 1990

Paris J, Frank H: Perceptions of parental bonding in borderline patients. Am J Psychiatry 146:1498–1499, 1989

Paris J, Zweig-Frank H: a critical review of the role of childhood sexual abuse in the etiology of borderline personality disorder. Can J Psychiatry 37:125–128, 1992

Paris J, Nowlis D, Brown R: Developmental factors in the outcome of borderline personality disorder. Compr Psychiatry 29:147–150, 1988

Regier DA, Boyd JH, Burke JD, et al: One month prevalence of mental disorders in the United States. Arch Gen Psychiatry 45:977–986, 1988

Robins LN: Deviant Children Grown Up. Baltimore, MD, Williams & Wilkins, 1966

Robins LN: Epidemiology of antisocial personality, in Psychiatry, Vol 3. Philadelphia, PA, JB Lippincott, 1989, Chap 19, pp 1–14

Robins LN, Helzer JE, Croughan J, et al: National Institute of Mental Health Diagnostic Interview Schedule: its history, characteristics, and validity. Arch Gen Psychiatry 38:381–389, 1981

Robins LN, Helzer JE, Ratcliff KS, et al: Validity of the Diagnostic Interview Schedule, Version II: DSM-III diagnosis. Psychol Med 12: 855–870, 1982

Salzman JP, Salzman C, Wolfson AN, et al: Association between borderline personality structure and history of childhood abuse. Compr Psychiatry 34:254–257, 1993

Schulz PM, Soloff PH, Kelly T, et al: A family history study of borderline subtypes. Journal of Personality Disorders 3:217–229, 1989

Snyder S, Goodpaster WA, Pitts WM, et al: Demography of psychiatric patients with borderline personality traits. Psychopathology 18:38–49, 1985

Spitzer R, Williams J, Gibbon M: Structured Clinical Interview for DSM-III-R, Version NP-V. New York, New York State Psychiatric Institute, Biometrics Research Department, 1987

Stone MH, Unwin A, Beacham B, et al: Incest in borderlines: its frequency and impact. International Journal of Family Psychiatry 9:277–293, 1988

Swartz M, Blazer D, George L, et al: Estimating the prevalence of borderline personality disorder in the community. Journal of Personality Disorders 4:257–272, 1990

Weiss DS: The IES revised. Paper presented at the annual meeting of the International Society for Traumatic Stress Studies, San Antonio, TX, October 1993

Westen D, Ludolph P, Misle B, et al: Physical and sexual abuse in adolescent girls with borderline personality disorder. Am J Orthopsychiatry 60:55–66, 1990

Zanarini MC, Frankenburg FR, Chauncey DL, et al: The Diagnostic Interview for Personality Disorders: interrater and test-retest reliability. Compr Psychiatry 28:467–480, 1987

Zanarini MC, Gunderson JG, Marino MF, et al: Childhood experiences of borderline patients. Compr Psychiatry 30:18–25, 1989a

Zanarini MC, Gunderson JG, Frankenburg FR, et al: The Revised Diagnostic Interview for Borderlines: discriminating BPD from other Axis II disorders. Journal of Personality Disorders 3:10–18, 1989b

Zweig-Frank H, Paris J: Parents' emotional neglect and overprotection according to recollections of patients with borderline personality disorder. Am J Psychiatry 148:648–651, 1991

Chapter 5

Relationship of Childhood Abuse and Maternal Attachment to the Development of Borderline Personality Disorder

Judith P. Salzman, Ed.D., Carl Salzman, M.D., and Abbie N. Wolfson, M.A.

Many contemporary researchers (Herman et al. 1989; Perry et al. 1990) assert that sexual abuse plays a major role in the genesis of borderline personality disorder (BPD). However, literature on both inpatient and outpatient samples (Briere and Zaidi 1989; Shearer et al. 1990) reveals that a history of sexual abuse, especially repeated abuse with multiple perpetrators, emerges almost invariably within the context of "family chaos" and "disrupted attachments" (Ludolph et al. 1990), "prickly and sticky" interpersonal attachments (Melges and Swartz 1989), parental neglect (Paris and Frank 1989), multiple caregivers, alcoholism, and/or evidence of affective instability (including both Axis I and Axis II disorders) among family members (Links et al. 1990).

A few studies, such as those of Zanarini et al. (1989a) and Ludolph et al. (1990), have attempted to compare the relative strength of a family climate of emotional violence and impaired attachments, as opposed to physical or sexual abuse per se, in predicting a diagnosis of BPD. In both these studies, results showed a stronger association between impaired family attachments, emotional violence, or neglect, and BPD than with the specific traumata of physical or sexual abuse. Others (Briere and Zaidi 1989; Links et al. 1990; Shearer et al. 1990; Westen et al.

71

1990) have suggested that childhood sexual abuse may be predictive of specific features of severely symptomatic borderline personality functioning, while not necessarily providing a comprehensive or general understanding of the etiology of this disorder. These features, as enumerated in the impulse section of the Diagnostic Interview for Borderlines (DIB; Gunderson et al. 1981), include "self-mutilation, manipulative suicide attempts, substance abuse, promiscuity and other forms of deviant sexuality, and other patterns of impulsive behavior, such as running away and assaults" (Westen et al. 1990, p. 60).

Similarly, Gunderson and Sabo (1993) urged clinicians to distinguish between shared diagnostic symptoms in BPD and PTSD, on the one hand, and clear differences, on the other hand, in etiology, duration, and frequency of these symptoms:

> It seems safe to conclude that the role of abuse in the pathogenesis of borderline psychopathology, although important, is neither specific nor sufficient. Borderline psychopathology arises out of a history in which abuse experiences join other factors to take part in shaping enduring aspects of the character. The abuse in such instances is symptomatic of more pervasive problems of enduring emotional neglect and extreme conflict with both parents. (p. 23)

Our thesis in this chapter, based on interview data with two nonclinical samples (Salzman 1988, Salzman et al. 1993), is that the variable of anxious attachment to mother outweighs that of abuse in the development of borderline personality—across the whole spectrum of that disorder, from the more withdrawn and isolated to the more impulsive and angry manifestations. In our discussion we present data on childhood abuse and attachment patterns from two nonclinical samples: one of female college undergraduates (Study 1), the other an adult volunteer sample of men and women recruited for a trial of fluoxetine (Study 2).

THEORETICAL BACKGROUND: ASSESSING ATTACHMENT IN ADOLESCENTS AND ADULTS

The potential usefulness of attachment theory for describing phenomena associated with BPD emerged initially in the context of a developmental study of adolescent attachment patterns (Salzman 1988). This study focused on attachment patterns in late-adolescent females, using a 2-hour semistructured interview. First piloted in 1982 with female high school students, the Adolescent Attachment Interview was developed during the same period as the Adult Attachment Interview (George et al. 1985). The Adolescent Attachment Interview was designed to record subjects' representations of their attachment experience (Salzman 1988, 1990). Like the Adult Attachment Interview, this approach is based on the assumptions that attachment representations, formed over time as inner psychological constructs, tend to be stable and that they correspond to the three major organizations of attachment experience identified by observations of infant behavior: secure, avoidant, and ambivalent.

The attachment interview protocol elicits a series of interlocking stories about a subject's primary attachments. The term *attachment figure* was defined for the purposes of the interview in accordance with criteria operationalized from Bowlby (1969, 1973, 1980) and Ainsworth et al. (1978): an individual to whom the subject has looked for nurturance, protection, availability, dependability, and empathic understanding, especially in times of stress or danger. The attachment figure's actual fulfillment of these criteria is seen to vary from one attachment group to another, and it is these variations that form the basis of subjects' differing internal representations of attachment.

Typically, a respondent who sees herself as securely attached according to this schema would describe freely seeking comfort and protection from an attachment figure, feeling soothed by interaction with that caregiver, having a clear sense of the caregiver's overall availability and behavioral consistency, and generally enjoying an experience of being understood by the caregiver. An avoidant respondent might share a sense of the caregiver's behavioral consistency, but this consistency would be described in negative terms: she cannot be counted on to soothe, protect, or understand. On the contrary, in this category, caregivers are seen as uniformly cold, hostile, and rejecting; respondents report "trying to stay out of her way as much as possible." An ambivalent subject, by comparison, would emphasize inconsistency in the attachment—an alternation between intense but often frustrating engagements with the mother and indifference or withdrawal on the mother's part. (See Table 5–1 for a more detailed explanation of attachment classifications.)

STUDY 1—AMBIVALENT ATTACHMENT AND BORDERLINE PHENOMENA: FINDINGS OF CLINICAL RELEVANCE FROM A NONCLINICAL SAMPLE

From a potential subject pool of 101 female college student volunteers, 41 interview subjects were selected in an approximation of stratified random sampling. Subjects' mean age was 20 years. Two were black, two Asian, and the rest white. No formal socioeconomic status (SES) measure was taken, but interview data suggest that the majority ranged from lower middle class to upper middle class.

It should be noted that in this sample of 41, subjects were chosen deliberately to provide approximately equal numbers in each of five attachment classifications: secure, ambivalent, avoidant, and two mixed groups—secure/ambivalent and secure/avoidant. The frequencies of interview subjects in these categories do not, therefore, correspond to those expected in a random sample. In true random samples, ambivalent and avoidant attachments, both considered forms of anxious attachment, generally constitute no more than 30%–34% of all subjects (Ainsworth 1978). True secure attachment, along with the two mixed groups delineated for Study 1, usually accounts for 66%–70% of attachments and, for purposes of our own data analysis, is defined as more securely attached than otherwise. Instead of true random sampling, therefore, an approximation of stratified random sampling was used to balance the numbers of interview subjects per attachment category.

All interviews were recorded and transcribed, then read by the first author and an independent rater to establish interview attachment classification. Raters also noted possible diagnostic evidence of either Axis I or Axis II disorders by DSM-III-R criteria (American Psychiatric Association 1987), based on subjects'

Table 5–1. Categories of attachment classification

Secure

Five critical variables reported present in attachment: nurturance, protection, availability, dependability, understanding. One caregiver also available as secure base from which to explore environment.

Avoidant

The five critical variables reported as deficient or absent. Caregiver described as frequently negative, critical, punitive, averse to physical contact. Subject often describes precocious attempts to establish complete self-reliance.

Ambivalent

Attachment described as intense but inconsistent with respect to the five critical variables. Frustrated longings, anxiety, and anger are subject's primary experiences in attachment.

Secure/Avoidant

Protection, availability, and dependability reported present in attachment. Emotional nurturance, physical comfort, and understanding absent. Love perceived as conditional on subject's achievements, independence.

Secure/Ambivalent

All five critical variables reported in early childhood, but attachment increasingly influenced by maternal anxiety and overprotection. By adolescence, subjects report struggle with separation/individuation. Depression frequently cited, as opposed to overt anger at caregiver.

---

self-reports. Interrater agreement on attachment classifications, derived from the attachment interview, was .92, using Cohen's kappa as a correction.

The clinical profile of ambivalent attachment delineated by interviews indicated major overlap between this attachment classification and vulnerability to BPD—specifically, to the more angry, impulsive, emotionally labile form of the disorder.

Table 5–2 details the diagnostic and attachment status of these young women. As can be seen, 11 of 41 subjects were classified as ambivalently attached. In this ambivalent group, 9 of 11 subjects reported at least 5 of the 8 requisite criteria for a diagnosis of BPD. Prominent among these were extreme interpersonal difficulties, intense, unmanageable attacks of anxiety or anger, rejec-

Table 5–2. Attachment classification and diagnosis in Study 1 subjects ($N = 41$)

Attachment classification	Diagnosis			
	BPD	Borderline trait	No diagnosis	Total
Secure	0	0	10	10
Secure/avoidant	0	0	7	7
Secure/ambivalent	0	1	5	6
Ambivalent	9	0	2	11
Avoidant[a]	0	0	7	7
Total	9	1	31	41

[a] As noted in the text, it was not possible to make accurate assessments of possible pathology among avoidant subjects in Study 1, because no formal diagnostic measures were employed. However, there were no clear manifestations of borderline symptomatology in this group's interview transcripts.

tion sensitivity, and unstable self-experience. Daughters offered numerous explicit examples of these phenomena and their origins in ongoing turbulent attachments to the mother. Their descriptions of these attachments included terms such as "push-pull relationship," "no-win love," "hot and cold" attachment, and "addictive love." These personal definitions indicate that *ambivalence* may be a misnomer in the research literature for an attachment experience that oscillates dramatically between love and hate but cannot truly encompass both feelings at any given time.

These subjects focused on their mothers' behavior as the source of all their own emotional turbulence, and they held their mothers responsible for their own personal distress. Throughout the interviews are descriptions of how mothers' perceived emotional lability affected the way daughters experienced attachment and how daughters at times had to accommodate to maternal demands for care, often at the daughters' own expense.

According to the daughters, attachment quality was most severely compromised by the intensity and unpredictability of the mothers' attacks on the daughters' self-esteem. Interview narratives reveal that mothers in the ambivalently attached group had appeared unable to provide steady, nurturant caregiving at any time within the subjects' memory. Instead, responses to their daughters' needs fluctuated according to the mothers' moods. These observations are consistent with those of Crittenden and Bonvillian (1984), Radke-Yarrow et al. (1985), Stern (1985), and Zahn-Waxler et al. (1984), who have noted the effects of maternal inconsistency or lability on infant and toddler attachment security.

In descriptions of their childhood, ambivalently attached subjects bore further witness to the psychologically disorganizing effects of maternal inconsistency. Their early memories portrayed a world where "things fall apart" and their mothers were too distracted or upset to offer comfort. Daughters commented that they were unable to hold their mothers' attention when they needed their mothers but that at other times their mothers' unsolicited responses would catch them unaware—often as a sudden outburst of rage. Conversely, at times when they fully expected their mothers to be angry or to discipline them, daughters would often be met instead with nonchalance or arbitrary leniency. One subject recalled such fluctuations as follows:

> I sat down on the sofa next to my mother and put my head in her lap, and it felt really nice. The next thing I knew, we were fighting, and we had one of the worst fights we have ever had in our lives. The next day, my mom is calling me at school: "I love you, I love you," and on the next day it would be over, until the next fight. Hot and cold, never anything in the middle.

Unlike avoidant attachments in this sample—where the mother was typically portrayed as predictably distant, cold, or unavailable—the bonds of ambivalent attachment appear to have been nourished by rare but delicious moments of contact, moments that stirred daughters' hopes of being understood. Unfortunately, that hope was never sustained. Instead, daughters in this study experienced an alternation between seduction and rebuff that perpetuated a deeply ambivalent but indissoluble bond. The paradoxical effect of such inconsistent or arbitrary maternal response was to perpetuate attachment-seeking behaviors in these young women. They appeared to behave as if hopelessly in thrall to their "bad objects" (Fairbairn 1946).

These observations have been partially supported by Kobak et al. (1993), who found a link between ambivalent attachment and "hyperactivating" interpersonal strategies that kept adolescents in a state of chronic dysfunctional anger toward parents. This pattern of hyperactivating was likewise found among subjects previously identified by Main and Goldwyn (1984) as "preoccupied with attachment," a category of anxious attachment and considered analogous to ambivalent attachment in infants.

From a psychodynamic viewpoint, it appears that ambivalent attachment stirred up intense frustrations and object hunger in this group of young women. Despite their intensity, however, ambivalent attachments were experienced as more negligent than overprotective. As in other studies of borderline personality pathology, the subjects' attachment experience reflects chaos, inconsistency, and anger alternating with indifference, as well as arbitrary limit setting (Gunderson et al. 1980). Owing to the detailed nature of subjects' reports, one can hear precisely how attachment to the mother may be simultaneously intense and oblivious to the child's needs. It is our hypothesis that this particular combination of experiences within attachment predisposes daughters to a more "hysterical"—that is, impulsive, acting-out—presentation of borderline pathology symptoms than to a more withdrawn or "schizoid" presentation.

It should be noted that with respect to abuse history, there were two reports of rape—one at age 5, the other in adolescence, both in the ambivalent attachment group—and that there were no other reports of sexual or physical abuse in the sample as a whole. The young woman reporting the childhood rape also described a suicide attempt and hospitalization during her first year at college. This pattern—an association between childhood abuse and symptom severity—is consistent with our thesis in this chapter: that one cannot explain borderline pathology overall by looking at abuse history, but that one may understand symptom severity in the light of past abuse.

Among securely attached subjects ($n = 10$), there was virtually no evidence of personality disorders, based on interview judgments. This group appeared emotionally resilient on both objective and interview measures of well-being, and their particular strength, in contrast to either of the anxious attachment groups, lay in their obvious social ease. They often cited confidence in their interpersonal skills as a trait shared with, and learned from, their mothers.

One might have expected at least some evidence of borderline pathology resulting from disturbed attachments in the avoidant attachment group ($n = 7$). However, unlike ambivalently attached subjects, who willingly offered detailed accounts of their attachment experience, avoidant subjects were not equally forthcoming or explicit, and it was therefore difficult to assess possible manifestations of pathology without the aid of specific diagnostic tools. Study 2, which established diagnosis first and then looked at attachment classifications, was intended in part to correct this methodological problem in Study 1.

STUDY 2—AVOIDANT ATTACHMENT AND BORDERLINE PHENOMENA: FINDINGS FROM AN ADULT VOLUNTEER SAMPLE

The second study gathered attachment interview data on 31 adult volunteers, all with borderline personality structure, who participated in a 13-week trial of fluoxetine compared with placebo. For this investigation, also using a nonclinical sample, subjects were diagnosed through two semistructured diagnostic interviews and a clinical interview applying DSM-III-R criteria. Unlike the first sample, which was deliberately constructed to include approximately equal numbers in five attachment categories, this second sample was recruited according to diagnosis only and without assessment of subjects' potential attachment classifications. It was assumed that the sample would include more anxiously attached (either avoidant or ambivalent) individuals than a random sample, but no effort was made to control for the distribution of attachment classifications, as in Study 1.

Subjects were recruited through newspaper advertisement for a study of the pharmacological treatment of volunteer subjects who had mild to moderate symptoms associated with BPD. As part of the screening for this investigation, subjects were asked about a history of physical or sexual abuse; questions were derived from Herman et al. (1989). Subjects who met DSM-III-R criteria for BPD, regardless of their history of abuse, then participated in the Structured Clinical Interview for DSM-III-R Personality Disorders (SCID-II) (Spitzer et al. 1987) and the Revised Diagnostic Interview for Borderlines (DIB-R) (Zanarini et al. 1989b). To meet criteria for a diagnosis of full BPD, subjects had to fit into one of the following two categories: 1) scoring 7 or greater on the DIB-R and 5 or greater on the BPD section of the SCID-II and also having a definite or probable DSM-III-R diagnosis of BPD from the clinical interview, or 2) scoring 8 or greater on the DIB-R and 4 or greater on the personality section of the SCID-II and also having a definite or probable DSM-III-R diagnosis of BPD from the clinical interview. To be diagnosed as having BPD traits, subjects had to meet the following criteria: 1) scoring 4–6 on the DIB-R and 4 or greater on the SCID-II and also having a definite DSM-III-R diagnosis of BPD from the clinical interview; or 2) scoring 7 or greater on the DIB-R and 4 or greater on the SCID-II and also having a definite DSM-III-R diagnosis of BPD from the clinical interview.

In addition to diagnosis, however, the investigators used certain exclusion criteria to ensure that this was a mildly to moderately symptomatic sample, albeit with clearly defined borderline pathology. In this respect, the second sample is comparable to the ambivalent attachment cohort in Study 1: little or no self-destructive behavior and no recent hospitalizations or suicidality.

Independent of sample selection and drug data gathering, two interviewers conducted attachment interviews with all 31 subjects accepted for the study. Three independent coders classified the interviews, using the same coding system as for Study 1; a high level of agreement was attained (.72, $P < .001$). One subject of 31 could not be reliably classified and was therefore dropped from attachment data analyses.

Data on childhood abuse history were gathered independently by clinical interview (at initial screening) and by attachment interview probes (adapted from Herman et al. 1989). Judgments of abuse history reported in attachment interviews were made independently by three clinicians, with unanimous agreement.

It was hypothesized, from results of the first study, that subjects with borderline personality diagnoses would report high frequencies of anxious attachment—most likely ambivalent attachment to the mother. Further, it was expected that the association between anxious attachment and BPD structure would be stronger than the association between abuse history and diagnosis.

As Table 5–3 shows, results confirmed these predictions. Breakdowns of attachment frequencies show only 2 out of 30 subjects classified as reporting strict secure attachment (omitting the 2 mixed groups), versus 5 classified as ambivalent and 12 classified as avoidant. These frequencies significantly differ from those expected in random samples ($\chi^2 = 50.5$, df = 2, P < .001). If one adds the two mixed groups (the 9 secure/avoidant subjects and the 2 secure/ambivalent subjects) to the strict secure classification to form a more securely attached group ($n = 13$), reported attachment frequencies (43% [13/30] secure versus 57% [17/30] anxious) still differ significantly ($\chi^2 = 22.3$, df = 2, P < .001) from those expected in random samples (66%–70% secure, 30%–34% anxious).

Contrary to expectations, the more common form of anxious attachment reported by participants in Study 2 was avoidant, not ambivalent, attachment. In fact, although virtually all subjects in Study 1 with borderline personality structure were classified as having ambivalent attachments, 12 of 30 subjects in Study 2 described avoidant attachments and only 5 in Study 2 described ambivalent attachments.

Table 5–3. Attachment classification and diagnosis in Study 2 subjects ($N = 30$)

| Attachment classification | Diagnosis | | |
	BPD	Borderline trait	Total
Secure	1	1	2
Secure/avoidant	5	4	9
Secure/ambivalent	2	0	2
Ambivalent	4	1	5
Avoidant	8	4	12
Total	20	10	30

Note. One out of 31 study subjects was dropped because raters could not agree on attachment classification.

Narrative data from the second study attests to avoidant sub-jects' own sense of withdrawal from overburdened, cold, or non-nurturant mothers. The following passages are representative of the collective experience of these 12 individuals:

> Oh yes. I mean, there was a suspicion in my mind that we were well taken care of. We weren't really physically or mentally abused, but there was no warmth there. It was sort of like we're not really wanted.
>
> Even now I watch her (the subject's mother) with my own baby and she really doesn't know what to do with her. Here's a little kid, let's not be cuddly. Instead it's poke, poke, pinch, pinch. She's hard. It's almost like she's afraid of the baby, she'll hurt it if she picks it up. Something will happen. So there's this distance. To this day, there's this distance (between us). I've given up. It's fine.
>
> She was very young—16—when she had me. She probably wasn't emotionally mature enough to be dealing with three little children . . . . I think she wanted to be there, meant to be there for me, but she didn't know how. And I didn't communicate to her what was really going on.

In contrast to observations from ambivalently attached subjects, the narratives quoted above reveal the paradigmatic experience of avoidant attachment: being on one's own much of the time, with a mother who was emotionally spent or otherwise unable to offer comfort or nurturance. Further, these avoidant subjects often cited being first- or lastborn in their families and remember their mother as being constantly busy with siblings, preoccupied with marital difficulties, and not "there" when needed. Unlike subjects with ambivalent attachments, those with memories of avoidant attachment did not persist in try-ing to engage with the mother, to win her affection or approval. In most cases, by middle childhood they concluded that the mother would never soothe, protect, or understand them. Often, they cited their own inability to express emotional needs as a partial reason for the failure to develop satisfactory attach-ments. In the words of one subject, "I usually kept very quiet, withdrawn, set back." And, from another, "[When I was upset,] I would go hide, either in the barn or in my room. I would just go away."

This attitude differs dramatically from that of ambivalent subjects in Study 1, who invariably blamed their mothers for their own distress within attachment. This basic difference in the experience of attachments continues into adolescence and adulthood, and it even reveals itself in the ways avoidant versus ambivalent subjects engaged with the interview process itself. Ambivalent respondents were emotionally expressive and detailed, and they wanted to be sure that interviewers knew the indignities they had suffered. In contrast, avoidant respondents tended to be terse and emotionally constricted and to have trouble elaborating their attachment memories. Explaining her inability to recall maternal attachment, one avoidant subject said that she had been a latchkey child from age 5 and that she could only remember unlocking the door to an empty house: "I don't remember her, I just remember" is the way she described the quality of attachment during childhood.

In this contrast between two groups with dissimilar profiles of borderline personality lies a possible understanding of how familial neglect may take quite different forms yet still contribute to the development of borderline structure. For young women in the first group, the mother was very much there, in the sense of expressing her own opinions and feelings, but rarely attuned to her daughter's needs. Daughters reported an insatiable and rarely satisfied emotional hunger, which felt to them like neglect. For subjects in the second study, neglect was more literal: for example, one subject had to be hospitalized for an extended time following an accident, and his mother simply could not care for him or visit him frequently. He did not blame her for this lapse; he simply accommodated to it, and his longings went underground.

With respect to one form of neglect—that of ineffective discipline—both groups did share a common memory. Most subjects, whether avoidant or ambivalent in their attachment experience, noted that caregivers did not set consistent limits for them as they were growing up. Discipline could be harsh, erratic, or absent, but it was not often the result of hovering or overprotection on the part of an anxious, concerned parent. These observations are consistent with findings of parental neglect reported by a number of other researchers, including Gunderson et al. (1980), Paris and Frank (1989), and Zweig-Frank and Paris (1991).

In summary, borderline subjects in Study 1 revealed a more consistent profile of emotional intensity, overt anger at caregivers, and dramatically difficult interpersonal relationships, characterized by extreme emotional need alternating with anger and contempt. In the second study, subjects had experienced more emotional withdrawal and isolation and held fewer expectations of what attachments might offer in the future. These subjects were more often accustomed to doing without nurturance from an early age, and many had the attitude of "false self-reliance" that Bowlby (1980) associated with avoidant attachment. In other words, subjects in the first study more nearly resembled the typical borderline personality with hysterical features, whereas those in the second study resembled those with a schizoid presentation. This distinction has been observed elsewhere (Johnson 1991) as being of possible prognostic value within the overall BPD classification.

DIFFERENCES BETWEEN STUDY SAMPLES

The results of Study 2 obviously cast doubt on the apparently exclusive linkage between ambivalent attachment and BPD suggested by Study 1. Possible reasons for the preponderance of ambivalent attachment in Study 1, compared with the greater proportion of BPD subjects classified as avoidant in Study 2, include the following:

1. As noted earlier, Study 1 did not use rigorous diagnostic methods. It is possible that among avoidant subjects in that sample, there may have been undiagnosed borderline pathology. Certainly, the 7 members of this group were less socially at ease than those in the secure attachment group, and 2 were frankly depressed, with some suicidal ideation. However, they did not report the same instability of self-image, turbulence in relationships, impulsive behavior, or intense anxiety and anger as those in the ambivalent attachment group. None met five out of eight DSM-III-R criteria for a diagnosis of BPD based on clinical interview data alone. Nevertheless, it may be that these 7 subjects, like the avoidant subjects in Study 2,

were inclined to be reserved and to minimize the depth of their distress to the interviewer. In both studies it would have been difficult, in fact, to diagnose borderline pathology in avoidant attachment from interview data alone. The addition of standard diagnostic instruments in Study 2 permitted investigators to identify borderline traits and disorder from a distance, as it were, and therefore enabled them to find evidence of this personality disorder among the avoidant subjects who were not talkers or complainers.

2. A second and more speculative reason for differences between samples lies in demographic characteristics. The Study 1 subjects with BPD or borderline trait tended to be younger and more affluent and to come from relatively smaller families (4 only children in this group of 10, and no subject with more than 2 siblings). Early divorce in their families of origin (5 of 10) was also common. These factors lent themselves, in daughters' opinions, to the development of intense, exclusive mother-daughter bonds and to the particular quality of object hunger that kept daughters coming back for more. One subject described the quasi-addictive quality of ambivalent attachment in the following manner: "I think my mother loves me, but she used her love to draw my love for her, to fill a void in her own life. We needed each other in that special way."

In contrast, subjects in Study 2 tended to come from larger, less affluent families. Few reported the intense, exclusive mother-child experience one might expect in a family consisting of a lonely divorced mother and her only daughter. Resources were stretched thinner in this sample, and, as noted earlier, there were more reports of genuine parental neglect, particularly emotional indifference or rejection, as opposed to gross physical neglect. It appears that this form of impoverished early experience, no less than more dramatic manifestations of overt rage, push-pull attachments, and violence, may quietly erode a developing sense of self, and of self in relationship. However, these individuals were clearly uncomfortable with calling attention to themselves, and they did not seek treatment easily. They were not accustomed to having others pay special attention to them.

The data from Study 2, then, suggest that these individuals with more avoidant or "schizoidal" borderline presentations might be underrepresented in research literature and might pass unnoticed, relative to the commoner acting-out borderline patient, in institutional settings.

RELATIONSHIP BETWEEN HISTORY OF CHILDHOOD ABUSE, DIAGNOSIS OF BORDERLINE PERSONALITY, AND SEVERITY OF BORDERLINE SYMPTOMS IN ADULT VOLUNTEERS

Of 31 subjects who completed the diagnostic phase of Study 2, only 6 (19.4%) revealed a history of physical or sexual abuse in childhood or early adolescence (Table 5–4). Two of the 6 reported both physical and sexual abuse, 1 reported physical abuse alone, and 3 reported sexual abuse alone. If one looks at full disorder compared with trait groups, one notes that 4 subjects reporting abuse were in the full-disorder group and 2 were in the trait group. This percentage of abused subjects in our sample differs from numbers reported by Herman et al. (1989)

Table 5–4.   Abuse history in Study 2 subjects

1. Subject was sexually abused by a neighbor at 4 or 5 years of age.

2. Subject was sexually abused by a male neighbor during early childhood over a 1.5-year period.

3. Subject was gang-raped at 14 years of age.

4. Subject underwent excessive corporal punishment by father until high school; subject stopped physical abuse by threatening to call the police.

5. Subject was sexually abused by a stranger one time between the ages of 5 and 7. Stranger was an older man who used candy to bribe the subject, then performed oral sex. Also, until subject was 8, mother disciplined by hitting with metal and wood shoehorn, leaving welts on one occasion.

6. Subject was beaten with electric appliance cords and hot irons during early childhood and was sexually abused by an aunt during early adolescence.

and Ogata et al. (1990). It more nearly resembles figures estimating abuse frequencies in nonclinical populations (Briere and Runtz 1988; Finkelhor 1979; Russell 1983) and therefore does not distinguish between individuals with a borderline diagnosis and those not carrying such a diagnosis.

We commented elsewhere (Salzman et al. 1993) that the discrepancy in the history of frequency of abuse between mildly symptomatic nonclinical populations and hospital or clinic populations suggests a spectrum of severity within the BPD diagnostic category. This view was supported by Westen et al. (1990) in their study of hospitalized BPD adolescents whose histories revealed a strong association between symptom severity and childhood abuse. Meissner (1984) also suggested a theoretical framework in which the BPD diagnosis represented a spectrum of psychopathology and symptom severity. In support of this theory, Koenigsberg (1982) showed that BPD inpatients, as compared with outpatient, have distinctly more severe manifestations of self-mutilation, substance abuse, and acting out within the therapeutic relationship. Our data suggest that along the severity spectrum, abuse is more often associated with severe rather than mild symptomatology. Three other studies (Links et al. 1990; Shearer et al. 1990; Westen et al. 1990) supported this relationship between severity of borderline symptoms and frequency of abuse history. Another three investigations (Briere and Zaidi 1989; Ludolph et al. 1990; Ogata et al. 1990) reported high rates of sexual abuse (52%–71%) among highly symptomatic psychiatric inpatients, suggesting that if one studies inpatient samples alone, one is likely to uncover high percentages of abuse histories. It is possible that the differences in frequency of abuse between our volunteer subjects and previously reported clinical samples resulted from missing information on abuse history taken from screening and attachment interviews. However, this seems unlikely, because the attachment interview permitted ample opportunity for subjects to retrieve and discuss traumatic memories.

With respect to drug effects in Study 2, the authors found no differences in fluoxetine response between abused and nonabused subjects, again suggesting that the variable of abuse in this sample did not play a significant discriminating role. In contrast, judging from improved DIB scores, it appears that attachment classification did interact with drug effect. Specifically, the subjects who responded best to fluoxetine were those identified as more securely attached (versus ambivalent or avoidant subjects (χ^2 = 10.4, df = 2, P < .006). If one omits the two mixed groups and compares only subjects classified as strictly securely attached with subjects classified as avoidant or ambivalent, the effect of fluoxetine is even more striking (χ^2 = 32.4, df = 2, P < .0001). In other words, the best drug response was in those subjects (n = 2) reporting truly secure attachment before treatment.

CONCLUSIONS

Our data indicate that an attachment framework may provide a more adequate basis for understanding borderline personality structure than simply noting the presence or absence of childhood abuse. In two separate studies, the variables of anxious attachment (either ambivalent or avoidant), coupled with a family climate of emotional instability/neglect, frequently accompanied the development of BPD symptomatology, whereas abuse per se (physical or sexual) appeared to be associated with symptom severity. In Study 1 (1988), which included 41 young women distributed across five attachment classifications, data analysis revealed almost complete overlap between a single attachment classification (ambivalent attachment) and diagnostic features of BPD. Nine of 11 young women in this category reported at least five out of eight DSM-III-R criteria for BPD, whereas only 1 other subject in the entire college sample appeared to have symptoms suggestive of borderline personality. In Study 2 (1993), borderline personality structure was diagnosed in all subjects (N = 31) before the study, but attachment frequencies were completely uncontrolled for. Here, results showed a strong association between avoidant attachment and borderline symptoms.

Thus, two studies posing quite different research questions showed significantly higher frequencies of anxious attachment (ambivalent or avoidant) among individuals with borderline personality structure than could be expected in random samples.

Both studies also showed stronger associations between border-line diagnosis and history of anxious attachment than between borderline diagnosis and a history of childhood abuse. Further, the variable that best explained differences between our two samples and borderline samples reporting much higher abuse frequencies was not overall diagnosis, but symptom severity. Among our own nonclinical groups there were no recent suicidal behaviors, no recent hospitalizations, and little or no self-destructive behavior (cutting, overdoses, or reckless or impulsive gestures) that would bring them to the attention of medical practitioners.

These findings raise the question of whether abuse is diagnostically specific for BPD, as opposed to other pathologies. The data suggest that anxious attachment to primary caregivers may be a substrate for the future development of characteristics of borderline personality; the addition of physical or sexual abuse may correlate with the severity of these characteristics. Future studies may clarify the relative weight of attachment, overall "family chaos," biological vulnerability, and abuse history in determining the development of borderline personality structure.

REFERENCES

Ainsworth M, Blehar M, Waters E, et al: Patterns of Attachment. Hillsdale, NJ, Lawrence Erlbaum, 1978, pp 59–64, 310–322, 343–356

American Psychiatric Association: Diagnostic and Statistical Manual of Mental Disorders, 3rd Edition, Revised. Washington, DC, American Psychiatric Association, 1987

Bowlby J: Attachment. New York, Basic Books, 1969

Bowlby J: Separation. New York, Basic Books, 1973

Bowlby J: Loss. New York, Basic Books, 1980

Briere J, Runtz M: Symptomatology associated with childhood sexual victimization in a nonclinical adult sample. Child Abuse Negl 12:51–59, 1988

Briere J, Zaidi LY: Sexual abuse histories and sequelae in female psychiatric emergency room patients. Am J Psychiatry 146:1602–1606, 1989

Crittenden PM, Bonvillian JD: The effect of maternal risk status on maternal sensitivity to infant cues. Am J Orthopsychiatry 54:250–262, 1984

Fairbairn WRD: Psychoanalytic Studies of the Personality. London, Routledge and Kegan Paul, 1946

Finkelhor D: Sexually Victimized Children. New York, Free Press, 1979

George C, Kaplan N, Main M: Adult Attachment Interview. Department of Psychology, University of California, Berkeley, CA, 1985

Gunderson J, Sabo AN: The phenomenological and conceptual interface between borderline personality disorder and PTSD. Am J Psychiatry 150:19–27, 1993

Gunderson JG, Kerr J, Englund DW: The families of borderlines. Arch Gen Psychiatry 37:27–33, 1980

Gunderson J, Kolb J, Austin V: The Diagnostic Interview for Borderline Patients. Am J Psychiatry 138:896–903, 1981

Herman JL, Perry JC, van der Kolk BA: Childhood trauma in borderline personality disorder. Am J Psychiatry 146:490–495, 1989

Johnson C: Psychodynamic Treatment of Anorexia Nervosa and Bulimia. New York, Guilford, 1991

Kobak RR, Cole HE, Ferenz-Gillies R, et al: Attachment and emotion regulation during mother-teen problem solving: a control theory analysis. Child Dev 64:231–245, 1993

Koenigsberg HW: A comparison of hospitalized and nonhospitalized borderline patients. Am J Psychiatry 139:1292–1297,1982

Links PS, Boiago I, Huxley G, et al: Sexual abuse and biparental failure as etiological models in borderline personality disorder, in Family Environment and Borderline Personality Disorder. Edited by Links PS. Washington, DC: American Psychiatric Press, 1990, pp 105–120

Ludolph PS, Westen D, Misle B, et al: The borderline diagnosis in adolescents: symptoms and developmental history. Am J Psychiatry 147:470–476, 1990

Main M, Goldwyn R: Predicting rejection of her infant from mother's representation of her own experience: implications for the abused-abusing intergenerational cycle. Child Abuse Negl 8:203–217, 1984

Meissner WW: The Borderline Spectrum: Differential Diagnosis and Developmental Issues. New York: Jason Aronson, 1984

Melges FT, Swartz MS: Oscillations of attachment in borderline personality disorder. Am J Psychiatry 146:1115–1120, 1989

Ogata SN, Silk KR, Goodrich S, et al: Childhood sexual and physical abuse in adult patients with borderline personality disorder. Am J Psychiatry 1147:1008–1013, 1990

Paris J, Frank H: Perceptions of parental bonding in borderline patients. Am J Psychiatry 146:1498–1499, 1989

Perry JC, Herman JL, van der Kolk, BA, et al: Psychotherapy and psychological trauma in borderline personality disorder. Psychiatric Annals 20:33–43, 1990

Radke-Yarrow M, Cummings EM, Kuczyniski L, et al: Patterns of attachment in 2- and 3-year olds in normal families and families with parental depression. Child Dev 56:884–891, 1985

Russell DEH: The incidence and prevalence of intrafamilial and extrafamilial sexual abuse of female children. Child Abuse Negl 7:133–146, 1983

Salzman JP: Primary attachment at adolescence and female identity: an extension of Bowlby's perspective (unpublished doctoral dissertation). Cambridge, MA, Harvard University, 1988

Salzman JP: Save the world, save myself, in Making Connections. Edited by Gilligan C, Lyons N, Hanmer T. Cambridge, MA, Harvard University Press, 1990, pp 110–146

Salzman JP, Salzman C, Wolfson AN, et al: Association between borderline personality structure and history of childhood abuse in adult volunteers. Compr Psychiatry 34:254–257, 1993

Shearer SL, Peters CP, Quaytman MS, et al: Frequency and correlates of childhood sexual and physical abuse histories in adult female borderline inpatients. Am J Psychiatry 147:214–216, 1990

Spitzer RL, Williams JBW, Gibbon M: Structured Clinical Interview for DSM-III-R Personality Disorders (SCID-II). New York, New York State Psychiatric Institute, Biometrics Research, 1987

Stern D: The Interpersonal World of the Infant. New York, Basic Books, 1985

Westen D, Ludolph P, Misle B, et al: Physical and sexual abuse in adolescent girls with borderline personality disorder. Am J Orthopsychiatry 60:55–66, 1990

Zahn-Waxler C, Chapman M, Cummings EM: Cognitive and social development in infants and toddlers with a bipolar parent. Child Psychiatry Hum Dev 15:75–85, 1984

Zanarini MC, Gunderson JG, Marino MF, et al: Childhood experiences of borderline patients. Compr Psychiatry 30:18–25, 1989a

Zanarini MC, Gunderson JG, Frankenburg FR, et al: The Revised Diagnostic Interview for Borderlines: discriminating BPD from other Axis II disorders. J Personality Disorders 3:10–18, 1989b

Zweig-Frank H, Paris J: Parents' emotional neglect and overprotection according to the recollections of patients with borderline personality disorder. Am J Psychiatry 148:648–651, 1991

Chapter 6

Relationship of Childhood Sexual Abuse to Dissociation and Self-Mutilation in Female Patients

Hallie Zweig-Frank, Ph.D., and Joel Paris, M.D.

D issociative phenomena may have an important relationship to traumatic events. The strongest evidence of this link is that patients with posttraumatic stress disorder (PTSD) have been shown to have unusually frequent dissociative symptoms (reviewed in Spiegel 1991). One theory used to explain this relationship is that dissociation develops as a defense against overwhelming threats, which allows the disowning of painful experiences through altered perceptions of the environment (Spiegel and Cardena 1991).

Because of the high frequency of trauma histories in borderline personality disorder (BPD) (see Zanarini, Chapter 1, this volume, for a review of the relevant research), it has been suggested that BPD itself is a form of chronic PTSD (Herman and van der Kolk 1987). In this view, the high levels of dissociation found in BPD are a consequence of trauma, and the presence of dissociative symptoms can be used as a marker for unrecognized trauma.

Research on dissociation has been aided by the use of standard instruments, such as the Dissociative Experiences Scale (DES) (Bernstein and Putnam 1986). Validation studies of this instrument (Carlson 1994) have shown that DES scores are par-

This research was supported by National Health Research Development Program, Canada Health and Welfare, Grant 6605-3486-CSA.

ticularly high in PTSD, are elevated in schizophrenia, and are generally higher in psychiatric patients than in nonpatients. Carlson factor-analyzed the DES into three scales, measuring disturbances of memory (amnestic), the capacity to ignore environmental stimuli (absorption), and changes in the perception of reality (depersonalization).

When patients with BPD are examined with semistructured interviews, they report high frequencies of dissociative symptoms (Zanarini et al. 1990a). The first purpose of our research was to determine whether this finding could be confirmed with the DES. In addition, we were interested in whether BPD is associated with any of the specific forms of dissociation described by Carlson.

As discussed in Paris and Zweig-Frank (Chapter 2, this volume), sexual abuse during childhood is particularly common in BPD, and there is a subgroup with severe childhood sexual abuse (CSA) in which abuse may play a particularly important role in the disorder. There have been several reports that dissociation in patients with personality disorders is linked with these histories of abuse (Chu and Dill 1990; Herman et al. 1989; Kirby et al. 1993; Ogata et al. 1990; Shearer 1994).

The second purpose of our research was, therefore, to determine whether dissociation in BPD is in fact linked with CSA. As discussed in Paris and Zweig-Frank (Chapter 2, this volume), community studies (Browne and Finkelhor 1986) showed that the parameters of CSA determine whether it leads to long-term sequelae. Our study was designed to determine whether any of these parameters has a stronger relationship to dissociation than does overall sexual abuse. In addition, we aimed to determine whether there was any association between dissociation in patients with personality disorders and other psychological risk factors, such as physical abuse, separation or loss, and problems in parental bonding.

Another phenomenon that could be associated with dissociation is self-mutilation (van der Kolk et al. 1991). Self-mutilation symptoms, particularly wrist slashing, are some of the most common clinical phenomena seen in BPD (Zanarini et al. 1990b). Clinical observations have suggested that borderline patients self-mutilate in part to obtain relief from dysphoric dissociative states (Leibenluft et al. 1987), and it has been proposed that self-mutilation in BPD is caused by traumatic experiences during childhood (Herman and van der Kolk 1987). There has also been one empirical study, in which nearly a third of the patients had BPD, that confirmed both of these relationships (van der Kolk et al. 1991). As with dissociation, it is possible that the parameters of childhood abuse could have a more specific relationship to self-mutilation than could an overall history of abuse. Moreover, the other psychological risk factors associated with BPD could interact with CSA in determining whether self-mutilation occurs.

Therefore, the third aim of the present study was to determine whether self-mutilation in patients with personality disorders is related to a history of sexual abuse and its parameters, other psychological risk factors, dissociation, diagnosis, or the interaction of all these variables.

METHODS

The overall design of the study is described in Paris and Zweig-Frank (Chapter 2, this volume). The following additional measures were used in the present report:

1. Dissociative Experiences Scale (DES): This widely used self-report scale (Bernstein and Putnam 1986) lists 28 items describing common dissociative experiences, each scored on a scale of 0–100. The total DES score is the mean of all 28 items. The three subscales developed by factor analysis—amnestic, absorption, and depersonalization (Carlson 1994)—were scored separately.
2. Self-mutilation: This was measured by item 72 on the Revised Diagnostic Interview for Borderlines (DIB-R) (Zanarini et al. 1989), which asks whether the patient has deliberately hurt herself without trying to kill herself any time in the last 2 years. Any positive answer to this question was scored as a history of self-mutilation. The total sample ($N = 150$) was divided into mutilators ($n = 48$) and nonmutilators ($n = 102$), and the BPD sample was also divided into mutilators ($n = 42$) and nonmutilators ($n = 36$).

RESULTS

Dissociation and BPD

The mean overall score and mean DES factor scores for the two diagnostic groups are presented in Table 6–1. The mean total DES score was significantly higher in the BPD group ($t = 5.5$, df $= 148$, $P < .0001$). The mean scores on all three DES factors were also significantly greater in the BPD sample: amnestic ($t = 4.3$, df $= 148$, $P < .0001$), absorption ($t = 5.6$, df $= 148$, $P < .0001$), and depersonalization ($t = 4.4$, df $= 148$, $P < .0001$).

Dissociation and Psychological Risk Factors

To examine specifically the relationship between dissociation and abuse, DES scores were submitted to a 2-way analysis of variance (ANOVA) with diagnosis and CSA as the independent variables. The main effect of diagnosis was highly significant [F $(1,146) = 28.3$, $P < .00001$]. Neither the main effect of CSA nor the 2-way interaction was significant.

A multiple regression was also carried out with the psychological risk factors (CSA, physical abuse [PA], separation or loss, and the four Parental Bonding Index [PBI] scales) as the independent variables and mean DES scores as the dependent variable (Table 6–2). None of the β scores was significant; the R^2

Table 6–1. Mean DES and DES factor scores in borderline and nonborderline subjects with personality disorders

Factor	BPD ($n = 78$)		Non-BPD ($n = 72$)	
	Mean	SE	Mean	SE
Total DES*	24.8	15.2	13.2	10.2
Amnestic factor*	13.4	14.6	5.3	7.4
Absorption factor*	36.2	20.4	19.6	14.5
Depersonalization factor*	7.7	17.1	7.6	10.1

Note. BPD, borderline personality disorder; DES, Dissociative Experiences Scale, SE, standard error.
*$P < .0001$.

was.04. The regression was repeated with diagnosis as an additional variable, and diagnosis was highly significant ($\beta = .41$, $P < .0001$, $R^2 = .19$). A multiple regression was carried out on each of the DES factor scores, and again there were no significant βs for any of the risk factors. These regressions were repeated with diagnosis entered, and again, in each case, only diagnosis was significant (amnestic factor: $\beta = .31$, $P < .0001$, $R^2 = .16$; absorption factor: $\beta = .43$, $P < .0001$, $R^2 = .19$; depersonalization factor: $\beta = .35$, $P < .0001$, $R^2 = .13$).

Additional analyses were then carried out to determine whether the parameters of CSA were related to DES scores. First, scores in subjects with caretaker CSA, noncaretaker CSA, and no CSA were compared in a 1-way ANOVA, and there were no significant differences. Second, a multiple regression of the CSA parameters (frequency, duration, age at onset, multiple perpetrators, fondling, genital fondling, oral sex, penetration, force, disclosure, ability to get help) on DES scores was carried out. None of the β scores was significant.

Table 6–2. Multiple regressions of psychological risk factors without and with diagnosis on mean DES scores in female patients with personality disorders ($n = 150$)

Variable	Risk factor (β)	Risk factor + diagnosis (β)
CSA	.05	.02
PA	.08	.03
Separation or loss	.07	.06
PBI scores		
Maternal affection	.06	.00
Maternal control	.03	.02
Paternal affection	.03	.03
Paternal control	.08	.10
BPD vs. non-BPD*	—[a]	.41
Multiple R	.20	.43
R^2	.04	.19

Note. BPD, borderline personality disorder; CSA, childhood sexual abuse; DES, Dissociative Experiences Scale; PA, physical abuse; PBI, Parental Bonding Index. [a]Empty cell, not applicable. *$P < .0001$.

Self-Mutilation and Psychological Risk Factors

Univariate Analyses

The frequency of CSA was greater in the self-mutilator than in the non-self-mutilator group (χ^2 = 4.3, df = 1, P < .05). There were no significant differences between these groups for the frequency of CSA by caretakers. There were also no significant differences between self-mutilators and non-self-mutilators for physical abuse, for separation or loss, or for the four PBI scales.

Multivariate Analyses

A logistic regression was carried out with CSA, PA, separation or loss, and the four PBI scales as independent variables and with self-mutilation as the dependent variable. None of these risk factors was significant.

Self-Mutilation, Dissociation, and Psychological Risk Factors

Univariate Analysis

The mean DES score in the self-mutilator sample was significantly higher than in the non-self-mutilator sample (t = −3.1, df = 148, P < .0002).

Multivariate Analyses

It was important to determine whether the findings in univariate analyses that mutilators had increased dissociation as well as increased CSA reflected the fact that both of these variables were highly associated with BPD. Therefore, multivariate analyses were conducted to clarify the relationship between dissociation, psychological risk factors, diagnosis, and self-mutilation.

First, a logistic regression was carried out in which psychological risk factors (CSA, PA, separation or loss, and the four PBI scales), DES scores, and diagnosis were the independent variables and self-mutilation was the dependent variable (Table 6–3).

This analysis showed that only diagnosis achieved significance (B = 1.2, $P < .001$, odds ratio = 3.4).

Second, to determine whether the borderline patients who self-mutilated ($n = 42$) differed from those who did not ($n = 36$) with respect to any of the risk factors (particularly CSA) and to dissociation, a logistic regression was carried out comparing these two groups, with psychological risk factors (CSA, PA, separation or loss, and the four PBI scales) and DES scores as the independent variables and self-mutilation as the dependent variable (see Table 6–3). None of the independent variables attained significance.

Finally, to examine whether any of the parameters of CSA were more strongly associated with self-mutilation than was overall CSA, a logistic regression was carried out on self-mutilation in abused subjects with all these parameters as the independent variables. The only significant variable was penetration ($\beta = .78$, $P < .02$, odds ratio = 1.3). However, when the regression was repeated with diagnosis as an additional independent variable,

Table 6–3. Logistic regression of psychological risk factors and DES scores on self-mutilation

Factor	All subjects ($n = 150$)		BPD only ($n = 78$)	
	β	SE	β	SE
CSA	.19	.23	.43	.28
PA	.06	.23	−.10	.31
Separation/loss	.32	.21	.32	.29
Maternal affection	.02	.02	.00	.03
Maternal control	.01	.02	.03	.03
Paternal affection	−.03	.02	.03	.03
Paternal control	−.03	.02	.02	.02
DES	.01	.01	.01	.02
Diagnosis	1.44	.36*		—
Constant	−1.39	.78	.04	1.2

Note. CSA, childhood sexual abuse; DES, Dissociative Experiences Scale; PA, physical abuse; SE, standard error.
*$P < .001$.

diagnosis was significant ($\beta = 1.7$, $P < .001$, odds ratio = 2.8), and penetration was no longer significant. An additional logistic regression compared borderlines who self-mutilated and borderlines who did not self-mutilate, with the parameters of CSA as independent variables. Again none of the parameters reached significance.

DISCUSSION

Our first question was whether DES scores are higher in borderline patients. We found that the mean total scores as well as the mean factor scores were all about twice as great in the BPD as in the non-BPD group. These results, therefore, confirm earlier reports, which used semistructured interviews (Zanarini et al. 1990a), finding that dissociative phenomena are more frequent in patients with BPD than in those with other personality disorders. There appears to be no particular form of dissociation associated with borderline pathology, but rather a broad range of dissociative phenomena, including amnestic tendencies, mental absorption, and depersonalization.

Our second question addressed the relationship between childhood sexual abuse and dissociation. We failed to find any such association in this sample of women with personality disorders. This negative finding came as a surprise to us. There were not even any trends in the direction of a positive relationship. Even finer-grained measures of CSA did not elicit any link with dissociation. For example, we did not find differences in DES scores between subjects with caretaker abuse and subjects with noncaretaker abuse. This finding stands in direct contrast to an earlier report (Chu and Dill 1990) in which only caretaker abuse was linked to dissociation. Nor did we find in a multiple regression that any of the parameters of CSA were related to DES scores. This finding stands in sharp contrast to a recent report (Kirby et al. 1993), in which more severe CSA was associated with higher DES scores.

We also failed to find that any of the other psychological risk factors had any relation to DES scores. In particular, we did not confirm earlier reports that childhood neglect is related to dissociation either in patients with personality disorders (van der Kolk et al. 1991) or in community populations (Nash et al. 1993). The discrepancy between our findings and those of previous reports could have several explanations. In one group of studies (Chu and Dill 1990; Kirby et al. 1993), diagnosis was not examined at all. In another report (Ogata et al. 1990), the authors commented that almost all their abused subjects had BPD and that therefore it was impossible to separate diagnosis from abuse history in relation to dissociation. In yet another study (Shearer 1994), only borderline subjects were studied. Our findings, however, stand in particular contrast to those of Herman et al. (1989), in which both abuse and diagnosis were found to be independently related to DES scores. It is possible that this particular discrepancy could be due to differences in methodology, because Herman et al. measured diagnosis as a continuous variable instead of comparing discrete diagnostic groups and did not examine sexual abuse separately, but only as part of a total trauma score.

The validity of our findings is supported 1) by the fact that this study was conducted on a larger sample than any previous report and 2) by a replication producing the same results on an equally large sample of men with borderline and nonborderline personality disorders (Zweig-Frank et al. 1994).

The absence of a relationship between CSA and levels of dissociation should be seen in the context of our findings that sexual abuse histories discriminated borderline from nonborderline personality disorders (see Paris and Zweig-Frank, Chapter 2, this volume). Although our findings point to CSA as a risk factor in some cases of BPD, they do not support the theory that dissociation in BPD is a part of a chronic posttraumatic syndrome. Finkelhor (1988) has proposed that the long-term effects of CSA need not necessarily involve dissociative mechanisms, but can be determined by cognitive mechanisms such as self-esteem regulation.

Since diagnosis was the only significant correlate of the level of dissociation, it might be argued that dissociation is an intrinsic aspect of BPD. The question of whether individual differences in the capacity to dissociate are under biological influence requires systematic genetic investigation. Two lines of indirect evidence bear on this hypothesis.

The first point is that the mean DES scores in BPD reported here are much lower than those previously reported for disorders uniquely related to psychological factors, such as PTSD (Bernstein and Putnam 1986; Carlson 1994). They are more similar to the scores found in schizophrenia (Bernstein and Putnam 1986), a disorder with a strong biological component, and in primarily neurological disorders such as temporal lobe epilepsy (Loewenstein and Putnam 1988).

The second point is that dissociative symptoms have been linked to hypnotizability (Carlson and Putnam 1989), and the capacity to enter a hypnotic trance has in turn been shown to be a function of a heritable personality dimension called "openness to experience" (Tellegen and Atkinson 1974; Tellegen et al. 1988). Thus, dissociative capacity among borderline patients may be related to a heritable personality trait that is independent of personal history.

Our third research question concerned whether abuse and dissociation are linked to self-mutilation in BPD. We again had primarily negative findings. Although in univariate analysis we did find significant relationships between CSA and self-mutilation, and between dissociation and self-mutilation, as had been found in an earlier study (van der Kolk et al. 1991), multivariate analyses revealed a more complex situation. Most of the self-mutilators had BPD, and it was these borderline subjects who had higher DES scores and more frequent histories of CSA. Thus the univariate relationships could all be accounted for by the presence of a borderline diagnosis. When all the psychological risk factors, DES scores, and diagnosis were examined multivariately in relation to self-mutilation in the total sample, only diagnosis remained significant. Moreover, none of the psychological risk factors (including CSA) or dissociation discriminated between borderline patients who self-mutilated and those who did not. Furthermore, although penetration was the only parameter of CSA that discriminated between borderlines who were self-mutilators and borderlines who were not, this relationship also disappeared when diagnosis was entered into the regression.

What these results do show is that, as in the case of dissociation, whereas sexual abuse discriminated borderline from nonborderline personality disorders, it did not discriminate borderlines who were self-mutilators from borderlines who were not. Nor did any of the CSA parameters, including penetration, discriminate between BPD patients who self-mutilated and those who did not. Since the difference between self-mutilating and non-self-mutilating borderline patients was not mediated by abuse variables and their parameters, or by levels of dissociation, the results do not provide support for the theory of Herman and van der Kolk (1987) that it is dissociation associated with a history of abuse that explains why borderline patients self-mutilate.

If dissociation and childhood sexual abuse do not account for self-mutilation in BPD, what other explanations could be considered? One possibility is that mutilating oneself might be accounted for in part by biological factors, such as trait impulsivity (Winchel and Stanley 1991). There is some empirical evidence for a relationship between impulsive aggression and reduced serotonergic activity (Coccaro et al. 1989). A recent study of patients with personality disorders showed that their degree of self-mutilation was negatively correlated with platelet imipramine binding (Simeon et al. 1992). It has also recently been shown that self-mutilation in BPD can in some cases be successfully treated by high doses of serotonin reuptake inhibitors (Markowitz 1993).

There is also some evidence that self-mutilation reflects social contagion (Walsh and Rosen 1985), a factor to which borderline patients could be particularly vulnerable. Therefore, some of the self-mutilating behavior observed in borderline patients could begin by imitation, rather than being specifically based on childhood experiences.

The main limitation of this study was our measure of self-mutilation, which was dichotomous rather than continuous, and which therefore did not reflect symptom severity. Although we might have found a relationship with sexual abuse if we had used a dimensional measure, the results here were not even at trend level. A second limitation is that the instrument we used assesses self-mutilation only in the last 2 years, not lifetime self-harm. (See Chapter 7 for a study that measured lifetime self-harm as a continuous variable, in which a significant relationship between both childhood abuse and neglect and self-harm was found.) A third limitation is that the measure of self-mutilation used here does not distinguish between different forms of self-harm, such as wrist slashing or head banging. Finally, as discussed in Paris and Zweig-Frank (Chapter 2, this volume), the psychological risk factors were measured retrospectively by self-report.

REFERENCES

Bernstein EM, Putnam FW: Development, reliability and validity of a dissociation scale. J Nerv Ment Dis 174:727–734, 1986

Browne A, Finkelhor D: Impact of child sexual abuse: a review of the research. Psychol Bull 99:66–77, 1986

Carlson EB: Studying the interaction between physical and psychological states with the Dissociative Experiences Scale, in Dissociation: Culture, Mind, and Body. Edited by Spiegel D. Washington, DC, American Psychiatric Press, 1994, pp 41–58

Carlson EB, Putnam FW: Integrating research in dissociation and hypnotic suggestibility. Dissociation 2:32–38, 1989

Chu JA, Dill DL: Dissociative symptoms in relation to childhood physical and sexual abuse. Am J Psychiatry 147:887–892, 1990

Coccaro EF, Siever LJ, Klar HM, et al: Serotonergic studies in patients with affective and personality disorders. Arch Gen Psychiatry 46:587–599, 1989

Finkelhor D: The trauma of child sexual abuse: two models, in Lasting Effects of Child Sexual Abuse. Edited by Wyatt GE, Powell GJ. Beverly Hills, CA, Sage, 1988, pp 61–82

Herman JL, van der Kolk BA: Traumatic antecedents of borderline personality disorder, in Psychological Trauma. Edited by van der Kolk BA. Washington, DC, American Psychiatric Press, 1987, pp 11–26

Herman JL, Perry JC, van der Kolk BA: Childhood trauma in borderline personality disorder. Am J Psychiatry 146:490–495, 1989

Kirby JS, Chu JA, Dill DL: Correlates of dissociative symptomatology in patients with physical and sexual abuse histories. Compr Psychiatry 34:258–263, 1993

Leibenluft E, Gardner DL, Cowdry RW: The inner experience of the borderline self-mutilator. Journal of Personality Disorders 1:317–324, 1987

Loewenstein RJ, Putnam, FW: A comparison study of dissociative symptoms in patients with complex partial seizures, multiple personality disorder, and posttraumatic stress disorder. Dissociation 1:17–23, 1988

Markowitz P: Longitudinal efficacy of SSRI in borderlines. Paper presented at the Third International Congress on the Disorders of Personality, Cambridge, MA, September 1993

Nash MR, Hulsey TL, Sexton MC, et al: Long-term sequelae of childhood sexual abuse: perceived family environment, psychopathology, and dissociation. J Consult Clin Psychol 61:276–283, 1993

Ogata SN, Silk KR, Goodrich S, et al: Childhood sexual and physical abuse in adult patients with borderline personality disorder. Am J Psychiatry 147:1008–1013, 1990

Shearer S: Dissociative phenomena in women with borderline personality disorder. Am J Psychiatry 151:1324–1328, 1994

Simeon D, Stanley B, Frances A, et al: Self-mutilation in personality disorders: psychological and biological correlates. Am J Psychiatry 149:221–226, 1992

Spiegel D, editor: Dissociative Disorders (section), in Review of Psychiatry, Vol 10. Edited by Tasman A, Goldfinger SM. Washington, DC, American Psychiatric Press, 1991, pp 143–280

Spiegel D, Cardena E: Disintegrated experiences: the dissociative disorders revisited. J Abnorm Psychol 100:366–378, 1991

Tellegen A, Atkinson G : Openness to absorbing and self-altering experiences ("absorption"), a trait related to hypnotic susceptibility. J Abnorm Psychol 83:268–277, 1974

Tellegen A, Lykken DT, Bouchard TJ, et al: Personality similarity in twins reared apart and together. J Pers Soc Psychol 45:1045–1050, 1988

van der Kolk BA, Perry JC, Herman JL: Childhood origins of self-destructive behavior. Am J Psychiatry 148:1665–1671, 1991

Walsh BW, Rosen PM: Self-mutilation and contagion: an empirical test. Am J Psychiatry 141:119–120, 1985

Winchel RW, Stanley M: Self-injurious behavior: a review of the behavior and biology of self-mutilation. Am J Psychiatry 148:306–317, 1991

Zanarini MC, Gunderson JG, Frankenburg FR, et al: The revised diagnostic interview for borderlines: discriminating BPD from other axis II disorders. Journal of Personality Disorders 3:10–18, 1989

Zanarini MC, Gunderson JG, Frankenburg FR: Cognitive features of borderline personality disorder. Am J Psychiatry 147:57–63, 1990a

Zanarini MC, Gunderson JG, Frankenburg FR, et al: Discriminating borderline personality disorder from other axis II disorders. Am J Psychiatry 147:161–167, 1990b

Zweig-Frank H, Paris J, Guzder J: Dissociation in male patients with borderline and non-borderline personality disorders. Journal of Personality Disorders 8:210–218, 1994

Chapter 7

Relationship Between Lifetime Self-Destructiveness and Pathological Childhood Experiences

Elyse D. Dubo, M.D., F.R.C.P.(C.), Mary C. Zanarini, Ed.D., Ruth E. Lewis, Ph.D., and Amy A. Williams, B.S.

Both self-mutilation and manipulative suicidal behavior are pathognomonic symptoms of borderline personality disorder (BPD) (Barrash et al. 1983; Frances et al. 1984; Zanarini et al. 1990). Self-destructive behavior as a whole is poorly understood, difficult to treat, and associated with a high degree of psychosocial morbidity. The literature addressing this phenomenon is largely based on heterogeneous groups of self-injurers that include patients with psychotic disorders, mental retardation, organic mental disorders, and various personality disorders (de Wilde et al. 1992; Favazza 1989; Favazza and Conterio 1988, 1989; Pattison and Kahan 1983; Rosenthal et al. 1972; Simeon et al. 1992; C. A. Simpson and Porter 1981; van der Kolk et al. 1991). Although the populations reported on probably encompass large numbers of patients with BPD, surprisingly few papers and very few controlled studies have focused on self-destructive behavior in exclusively borderline samples (Dulit et al. 1994; Gardner and Cowdry 1985; Leibenluft et al. 1987; Perry 1989; Russ et al. 1993; Schaffer et al. 1982; Shearer et al. 1988; M. A. Simpson 1977; Soloff et al. 1994; Stone 1987; van der Kolk et al. 1991).

Deliberate self-injurious behavior and true suicidal acts have been distinguished in the literature as separate clinical problems

Supported in part by National Institute of Mental Health grant MH 47588.

(Gardner and Cowdry 1985; Leibenluft et al. 1987; Pattison and Kahan 1983; Stone 1987). Suicidal behavior is more common after midlife; during this period, completed suicides are more frequent in males. Habitual self-mutilation, however, characteristically begins in late adolescence, often continues for decades, and occurs predominantly in females (Favazza and Conterio 1988, 1989; Pattison and Kahan 1983). Self-mutilation frequently involves numerous episodes of self-harm, which are often ritualized and employ multiple methods of low lethality. This behavior is commonly associated with impulsivity, and absence of pain has frequently been reported (Favazza 1989; Favazza and Conterio 1988, 1989; Gardner and Cowdry 1985; Leibenluft et al. 1987; Pattison and Kahan 1983; M. A. Simpson 1977). Chronic cutting and self-inflicted cigarette burns to the wrists, arms, or other parts of the body are the most common means, but other methods include self-hitting and scratching, interfering with wound healing, hair pulling, and bone breaking (Favazza and Conterio 1988, 1989; Gardner and Cowdry 1985; C. A. Simpson and Porter 1981).

Unlike suicidal behavior, self-mutilation is associated with relief from intolerable affects, such as despair, anxiety, rage, loneliness, and self-hatred, and it has frequently been described as a desperate recourse to alleviate feelings of depersonalization (Favazza 1989; Favazza and Conterio 1988, 1989; Pattison and Kahan 1983; Rosenthal et al. 1972; M. A. Simpson 1977; C. A. Simpson and Porter 1981). These dysphoric affects are often precipitated by a crisis in a significant personal relationship involving real or perceived abandonment, rejection, or neglect (Leibenluft et al. 1987; Rosenthal et al. 1972; Rosenthal and Rosenthal 1984; M. A. Simpson 1977; C. A. Simpson and Porter 1981). In this context, self-mutilation, unlike true suicidal acts, frequently serves as a means of communicating to significant others internal distress that cannot be put into words (Leibenluft et al. 1987).

Several authors have reported on the childhood experiences characteristic of patients who chronically inflict injury on themselves or make suicide attempts. Significantly related childhood factors have included parental neglect (Bach-y-Rita 1974; Rosenthal and Rosenthal 1984; C. A. Simpson and Porter 1981; van der

Kolk et al. 1991), parental loss or separation (Carroll et al. 1980; C. A. Simpson and Porter 1981; van der Kolk et al. 1991), early physical trauma and repeated surgery (Rosenthal et al. 1972), physical abuse (Carroll et al. 1980; Favazza 1989; Green 1978; Grunebaum and Klerman 1967; Rosenthal and Rosenthal 1984; Roy 1978; C. A. Simpson and Porter 1981; van der Kolk et al. 1991), and sexual abuse (de Wilde et al. 1992; Russ et al. 1993; C. A. Simpson and Porter 1981; Stone 1987; van der Kolk et al. 1991).

In a consecutive series of 66 female inpatients, Bryer et al. (1987) found that subjects with a childhood history of sexual abuse were not only more likely to have BPD but exhibited significantly more suicidal behavior than the nonabused group. Links et al. (1990) studied a group of 88 inpatients with BPD and found that those with a history of sexual abuse evidenced more self-mutilation and other physically self-damaging behaviors, substance abuse, depersonalization, and derealization than did nonabused borderline subjects. Westen et al. (1990) compared histories of childhood trauma in adolescent inpatient girls with BPD and in control subjects. They found a significant association between scores on the Impulse section of the Diagnostic Interview for Borderlines (DIB) (Gunderson et al. 1981) and histories of sexual abuse. This relationship was true for both the borderline group and the control subjects. The behaviors rated in the Impulse section include self-mutilation and manipulative suicide attempts. Westen et al. found no relationship between life-threatening suicide attempts and either sexual or physical abuse. Russ et al. (1993), studying a sample of 27 female adult inpatients with BPD and chronic self-destructive behavior, found that those who did not experience pain during self-harm (13 patients) were more impulsive, made more suicide attempts, experienced more dissociation, and had a higher prevalence of childhood sexual abuse than was true for the subjects who did experience pain. These preliminary findings suggest a possible link between childhood sexual abuse, dissociation, analgesia, and a more malignant course of self-destructive behavior.

Only one study has looked systematically at the relationship between a variety of harmful childhood factors and self-destructive behavior. Van der Kolk et al. (1991), using both historical and prospective data for 74 subjects with personality disorders or bipolar II disorder, found that histories of childhood trauma, particularly sexual abuse, and histories of childhood neglect were highly significant predictors of chronic suicide attempts, cutting, and other self-injurious behavior. The authors reported that chronic suicide attempts were most strongly associated with histories of childhood sexual abuse, whereas chronic cutting was most strongly associated with histories of childhood neglect. Because in their study the borderline diagnosis was the only diagnosis significantly associated with physically self-destructive behavior, their findings may well be specifically related to patients with BPD.

The study described below builds on this work. It aimed both 1) to define the lifetime patterns of self-destructive behavior in criteria-defined patients with BPD compared with control subjects who had near-neighbor Axis II disorders and 2) to relate these patterns to the subjects' pathological childhood experiences.

METHODS

All subjects were inpatients drawn from a larger sample that was part of the DSM-IV Axis II field trials. The methodology of this study is basically the same as that described by Zanarini et al. (Chapter 3, this volume). The one exception was that we also administered the Lifetime Borderline Symptom Index (LBSI)—a structured instrument we created for this study, based on the symptom categories of the Revised Diagnostic Interview for Borderlines (DIB-R) (Zanarini et al. 1989b). This instrument rates the age at onset, duration, severity, and number of episodes of a variety of key borderline symptoms over a patient's lifetime. For most items in this instrument, continuous variables are generated.

The means of continuous variables were compared by using Student's t test. Categorical variables were compared by using χ^2 analyses with Yates correction for continuity. Multiple regression analyses were used to assess the relationship between the various childhood factors and various aspects of self-destructive behavior.

RESULTS

The subjects were 42 patients who met criteria for BPD and 17 control subjects with near-neighbor Axis II disorders. In the borderline group, there were 30 women (71.4%) and 12 men (28.6%); the control group consisted of 10 (58.8%) women and 7 (41.2%) men. The age range of the borderline group was 18–60 years, and that of the control subjects was 20–57 years. Mean ages were 31.7 years for the borderline group and 35.9 years for the control group. There were no significant differences in sex distribution or mean age between the two groups.

Thirty-three patients (78.6%) with BPD reported histories of self-mutilation, whereas no control subjects reported this type of behavior. Thirty-four (80.9%) of the borderline patients and 5 (29.4%) of the control subjects reported histories of suicide attempts.

Self-Mutilation

The age at onset of self-mutilative behavior ranged from 4 to 47 years. The mean age at onset was 20.7 years (± 10.1). The majority (26; 61.9%) of patients with BPD began mutilating themselves in adolescence or adulthood. Smaller numbers began in early childhood (2; 4.8%) and latency (5; 11.9%). The prevalence of self-injurious behavior in the borderline group increased steadily from early childhood to adulthood (2, or 4.8%, in early childhood; 7, or 16.7%, in latency; 16, or 38.1%, in adolescence; and 29, or 69.0%, in adulthood). This is in part due to the increased number of subjects beginning to self-mutilate in adolescence and adulthood, but it also reflects the continuation of this behavior in the patients who began at a young age. Reported number of lifetime instances of self-mutilative efforts ranged from 1 to 3,000. Mean number of instances was 233.2 (± 548.2). Only 3 (7.1%) of the borderline patients self-mutilated once or twice; 17 (40.5%) engaged in 50 or more episodes of self-mutilative behavior over a lifetime. Duration of self-mutilative behavior ranged from 1 month or less to 552 months (46 years). The mean duration was 107.8 months (± 123.7), or 9 years.

Suicide Efforts

Thirty-four of 42 patients with BPD (80.9%) and 5 of 17 control subjects (29.4%) engaged in suicidal behavior. There was no significant difference in mean age at onset of suicide efforts between groups: mean age at onset was 21.4 years (± 9.6) for the borderline group and 22.8 years (± 9.0) for the control group. Age at onset ranged from 6 to 48 years for the borderline subjects and from 16 to 35 years for the control subjects. In the borderline group, 11.9% (5) began their suicide efforts in latency. Onset of suicidal behavior occurred in increasing numbers through adolescence (21.4%, or 9) and adulthood (47.6%, or 20). In contrast, patients in the control group did not begin their suicidal behavior until adolescence (17.7%, or 3), and fewer began in adulthood (11.7%, or 2). For the borderline group, the prevalence of suicidal behavior during each period followed a pattern similar to that seen for self-injurious behavior—that is, there was a steady increase in numbers over adolescence and adulthood (30.9%, or 13, and 71.4%, or 30, respectively). This pattern reflects both the increasing number of subjects newly making suicide attempts as well as the tenaciousness of their suicidal behavior. In contrast, the prevalence for the control group was the same during adolescence as adulthood (17.6%, or 3), reflecting the shorter duration of their suicidal behavior and the decline in onset of this behavior after adolescence. Patients with BPD made significantly more suicide attempts over their lifetime than patients in the control group. The mean number of instances for the borderline group was 20.1 (± 46.6), compared to a mean of 2.4 (± 1.3) for the control group ($P < .03$). Borderline patients made 1–200 attempts, whereas control subjects made only 1–4 attempts; 44% of the borderline group made 5 or more suicide attempts. There was no significant difference in mean duration of suicidal behavior between groups. Mean duration of suicidal activity for the borderline group was 102.6 months (± 121.8), or 8.6 years. Duration ranged from 1 month or less to 504 months (42 years). For the control group, mean duration of suicidal activity was 56.2 months (± 122.9), or 4.7 years; the duration ranged from 1 month or less to 276 months (23 years).

Super Self-Destructiveness

A subgroup of patients with BPD engaged in extremes of self-mutilative and/or suicidal behavior. We defined *super self-mutilators* as those who had made 50 or more self-mutilative efforts in their lifetime and *super suicide attempters* as those who had made 5 or more attempts in their lifetime. In this sample of borderline patients, 40.5% (17) were super self-mutilators and 42.9% (18) were super suicide attempters. All the borderline subjects who began to self-mutilate in early childhood were found in the extreme group, as were the borderline subjects who made the earliest suicide attempts. Sixty-five percent (11) of borderline subjects who engaged in extreme self-mutilative behavior also engaged in extreme suicidal behavior, clearly forming the subgroup with the highest morbidity and the highest risk of mortality (26.2% of the entire borderline sample, or 11 subjects).

Self-Destructive Behavior and Childhood Factors

The relationship between self-destructive behavior and 12 childhood factors was examined in multiple-regression format: caretaker emotional abuse, verbal abuse, and physical abuse; sexual abuse by caretakers; sexual abuse by noncaretakers; caretaker physical neglect; emotional withdrawal, inconsistent treatment, emotional denial, and lack of a real relationship with a caretaker; parentification of the patient by a caretaker; and failure to protect by a caretaker.

It was revealed by χ^2 analyses that when childhood factors were viewed as categorical variables, no factor was more frequently associated with the borderline group than with the control subjects. This can be seen as a reflection of the degree to which the control subjects with Axis II disorders were very near neighbors to this acutely ill inpatient borderline group.

Self-Destructiveness and Childhood Abuse

Abusive childhood experiences were considered first. Multiple regressions were performed to determine the influence of childhood verbal, emotional, physical, and sexual abuse on the onset, lifetime number of episodes, and duration of self-mutilative and suicidal efforts in patients with BPD. Subject's sex was also controlled for. The significant findings can be seen in Table 7–1.

Age at onset of self-mutilative behavior was not related to any of the abuse variables. Lifetime number of self-mutilative efforts was significantly related to caretaker sexual abuse ($P < .05$). Lifetime duration of self-mutilative behavior was also significantly associated with sexual abuse by caretakers ($P < .05$).

Subject's sex predicted age at onset of suicidal behavior—that is, female subjects began to make suicide efforts at an earlier age than their male counterparts ($P < .05$). There was no relationship between any of the abuse variables and number of suicide efforts. However, lifetime duration of suicidal behavior was strongly associated with caretaker sexual abuse ($P < .005$).

Self-Destructiveness and Childhood Abuse and Neglect

Table 7–2 shows the significant results of the childhood abuse and neglect variables considered together in multiple-regression format for patients with BPD. For self-mutilative behavior, childhood sexual abuse no longer appeared to be the most important factor, and several aspects of childhood neglect gained significance. Emotional withdrawal by a caretaker predicted age at onset of self-mutilative behavior ($P < .05$). There remained

Table 7–1. Multiple regression analyses of childhood abuse variables and self-destructive behavior (BPD group)

Outcome variable	Childhood abuse variable	P
Self-mutilation		
Age at onset	—	—
Number of instances	Sexual abuse by caretaker	$< .05$
Duration	Sexual abuse by caretaker	$< .05$
Suicide efforts		
Age at onset	—	—
Number of instances	—	—
Duration	Sexual abuse by caretaker	$< .005$

Note. Empty cells indicate nonsignificant results.

a weaker but significant relationship between lifetime number of instances of self-mutilation and caretaker sexual abuse ($P < .05$). Duration of self-injurious behavior was significantly related to failure to protect by a caretaker ($P < .05$) and inconsistent treatment by a caretaker ($P < .005$).

Age at onset of suicidal behavior remained associated with subject's sex. Lifetime number of suicidal efforts was not related to any of the abuse or neglect variables. Lifetime duration of suicidal behavior continued to be significantly related to sexual abuse by caretakers.

The childhood experiences of the control subjects were also explored by using a multiple regression format; the significant findings are presented in Table 7–3. In contrast to the borderline group, the abuse variables were not significantly related to suicidality. Three neglect variables, however, were significantly related to suicidal behavior in the control group: emotional withdrawal and emotional denial by a caretaker were associated with lifetime number of suicide efforts ($P < .05$ and $P < .001$ respectively), and lack of a real relationship with a caretaker was associated with lifetime duration of suicidal behavior ($P < .001$).

Table 7–2. Multiple regression analyses of childhood abuse/neglect variables and self-destructive behavior (BPD group)

Outcome variable	Childhood abuse/ neglect variable	P
Self-mutilation		
Age at onset	Caretaker emotional withdrawal	< .05
Number of instances	Sexual abuse by caretaker	< .05
Duration	1. Failure to protect by caretaker	< .05
	2. Inconsistent treatment by caretaker	< .05
Suicide efforts		
Age at onset	—	—
Number of instances	—	—
Duration	Sexual abuse by caretaker	< .005

Note. Empty cells indicate nonsignificant results.

DISCUSSION

This study revealed several significant findings regarding the lifetime patterns of self-destructive behavior in patients with BPD and the role of childhood sexual abuse and neglect in its development.

High Levels of Self-Harm

We found that as a group the borderline patients reported a tremendous amount of self-harm. Self-mutilation was seen exclusively in the borderline subjects, reflecting the discriminating power of this symptom. Approximately 79% of subjects with BPD reported a history of self-mutilative behavior, which was typically chronic and highly repetitive. About the same percentage, 81%, of borderline patients gave a history of suicide attempts, compared to only 29% of control subjects. Borderline subjects characteristically made repeated suicide attempts, and they reported a significantly greater number of suicide efforts over their lifetime than did the control subjects. Our results confirmed previous reports that self-destructive behavior is highly discriminative of BPD (Barrash et al. 1983; Frances et al. 1984; Zanarini et al. 1990) and demonstrated empirically that this behavior is characteristically severe and enduring.

Table 7–3. Multiple regression analyses of childhood abuse/neglect variables and self-destructive behavior (OPD group)[a]

Outcome variable	Childhood abuse/ neglect variable	P
Suicide efforts		
Age at onset	—	—
Number of instances	1. Caretaker emotional withdrawal	< .05
	2. Caretaker emotional denial	< .001
Duration	Lack of a real relationship with caretaker	< .001

Note. Empty cells indicate nonsignificant results.

Childhood-Onset Self-Destructive and Super Self-Destructive Subgroups

The results of this study also illustrate that there is a subgroup of borderline patients who begin to injure themselves and/or attempt suicide at a very young age. Consistent with previous reports, we found that the onset of self-destructive acts most commonly occurred in late adolescence and early adulthood (Favazza and Conterio 1988, 1989; Pattison and Kahan 1983). Approximately 5% of borderline subjects (2), however, began to self-mutilate in early childhood (0–5 years), and nearly 12% (3) began to make suicide attempts as early as latency (6–12 years). In all cases, those who started very young continued their self-injurious behavior into adulthood. This group deserves further study to elucidate what factors are specifically related to childhood onset of self-destructive behavior.

Our findings also bring to light that within the borderline population is a subgroup of patients who are extraordinarily self-destructive. Subjects who began to self-harm at the earliest ages tended to fall into this category, but it also included subjects who became self-destructive in adolescence and adulthood. Whereas previous studies have rated the presence or absence of self-injurious behavior, we used an instrument rating (albeit retrospectively) the lifetime number of self-destructive episodes. We found that 40.5% (17) of our borderline subjects were extreme self-mutilators, having engaged in 50 or more episodes of self-mutilation in their lifetime. We also identified a subgroup of extreme suicide attempters. Fully 42% (18) of the borderline group made 5 or more suicide attempts in their lifetime. There was significant overlap between these two subgroups: 65% (11) of borderline subjects who engaged in extreme self-mutilative behavior also engaged in extreme suicidal behavior. More than one-quarter of the entire borderline sample (11) met criteria for this super self-destructive subgroup. This probably reflects the overall high acuity of our inpatient sample, and it may be an overestimate for less disturbed populations of borderline patients.

Nonetheless, this group presents a serious clinical problem associated with severe morbidity and greatly increased risk of mortality. It may be that these patients were subject to more profound emotional neglect and a greater degree of family chaos (see Zanarini et al., Chapter 3, this volume). They may have been more severely sexually abused or abused at an earlier age; van der Kolk et al. (1991) found that the earlier any trauma occurred, the more self-destructive behavior reported, especially cutting. Numerous studies have shown a heightened risk of BPD in the first-degree relatives of borderline patients (see Gunderson and Zanarini 1989 for a review of this topic). It is possible that severely self-destructive borderline patients are more likely to be the product of poorly modulated, impulsive, and self-destructive borderline parents. If this is the case, extreme self-destructiveness may be both inherited genetically and engendered environmentally through pathological parenting and traumatic childhood experiences. These borderline patients may be different temperamentally, or they may have a particular biological predisposition to self-destructive behavior. They may be similar to the borderline patients that Andrulonis et al. (1981) described as having underlying neurological abnormalities associated with possible limbic system dysfunction and episodic dyscontrol.

Childhood Factors

The central purpose of our study was to examine the role of childhood factors in the development of self-destructive behavior in borderline patients. Our results lend additional support to previous observations that both caretaker sexual abuse and caretaker emotional neglect play an important role in the etiology of self-harm. Our findings demonstrate that when the influence of childhood abuse is examined separately from childhood neglect, its role in the etiology of self-destructive behavior in BPD appears of singular importance. However, when the effects of childhood sexual abuse are viewed within the context of the emotionally detached and nonprotective relationships in which it typically occurs, the neglectful features of the borderline patient's familial environment gain etiological importance. When we looked first at the effects of various types of childhood abuse on the development of self-destructive behavior, we found that sexual abuse by caretakers was highly predictive of both self-mutilative and suicidal behavior. This is consistent with the numerous reports in the literature that have cited the high inci-dence of suicide attempts and other forms of self-destructive behavior among victims of incest (Browne and Finkelhor 1986). When we considered the effects of childhood abuse and neglect together, a more complex picture developed. Although parental sexual abuse continued to strongly predict suicidal behavior, parental emotional neglect emerged as the strongest predictor of self-mutilative behavior.

These findings confirmed the observations reported by van der Kolk et al. (1991) and suggest that lack of early parental emotional responsiveness and protection play an important role in the development of affective dysregulation leading to chronic self-mutilation in patients with BPD. It appears that parental sexual abuse may increase the severity of self-mutilation and drive chronic suicidal behavior. Overall, our results underscored the role of both parental sexual abuse and emotional neglect in the etiology of self-destructive be-havior in borderline patients and highlighted the importance of considering the effects of sexual abuse within its environ-mental context.

A surprising finding was that when we viewed the childhood experiences of our subjects as categorical variables, the border-line group did not appear to have more trauma or neglect in their histories than did the control group. This is inconsistent with previous studies reporting a higher prevalence of child-hood histories of sexual abuse and neglect in borderline cohorts than in other populations. A possible explanation is that our control group was largely composed of patients from the dra-matic cluster, including many with antisocial personality disor-der, and many who just missed meeting our research criteria for BPD. Our findings indicate that it may be the interaction of particular childhood variables, or the additive effect, that is im-portant for the development of certain types of borderline symp-toms. How abuse and neglect actually relate to causality is uncertain. In addition to their possible direct effects on develop-ment, it is also plausible that problems with impulsivity and poor affect tolerance are being passed down genetically, as reflected in the existence of these problems in the abusive, neglectful parents. In addition, it may be that as a result of constitutional factors, borderline patients respond to their experiences differently than do other types of patients who have endured similar experiences. Prospective studies of abused and neglected children are needed in order to determine which factors specifically influence the development of BPD.

Finally, whereas for the borderline subjects an admixture of sexual abuse and emotional neglect was related to suicidality, we found that for the control subjects only neglect was significantly associated with a history of suicide attempts. This further supports the notion that parental validation of feelings and experiences is critical to the development of affective self-regulation.

Symptoms and Course

Although our study was limited by the retrospective nature of the data, the relatively small sample size, and the possibility that findings based on an inpatient population of borderline patients may not be generalizable to a less disturbed outpatient population, our results suggest that 1) there may be subgroups of borderline patients who differ in symptom presentation and course and 2) these differences may, at least in part, be related to their childhood experiences. We believe the patients' reports of their traumatic childhood experiences to be valid; they were given in rich detail, and the patients usually presented their material with a great deal of anxiety, sadness, and affective lability. Clearly, large prospective studies are needed to clarify further which environmental, constitutional, and/or biological factors account for subsyndromal differences and to determine the most effective early interventions for at-risk children.

Self-Harm as Form of Communication

Self-destructive behavior is one of the most difficult problems for clinicians to understand and treat. Complicated emotional responses, involving some combination of helplessness, horror, rage, guilt, disgust, and sadness, are commonly invoked in the treaters of patients who repeatedly harm themselves (Frances 1987). Difficulty in managing this behavior frequently leads to a major impasse in the treatment, which can result in its ending, or, in the worst-case scenario, in the death of the patient (Gunderson 1984). The literature addressing the phenomenology and treatment of patients with BPD, and the problem of self-destructive behavior in general, includes efforts to explain this behavior in intrapsychic, psychodynamic, developmental, and biological terms. Treatment approaches described in the literature have been equally varied. Perry (1989) studied intrapsychic conflicts in patients with BPD and found that separation-abandonment conflict, object hunger, and conflict regarding the experience and expression of emotional needs and anger were significantly correlated with self-injurious behavior. This fits well with our observation that lack of protective, securely attached relationships with caregivers appears to be etiological in the development of self-mutilative behavior in this group.

Several authors have noted the communicative value of self-destructive behavior in borderline patients (Gardner and Cowdry 1985; Gunderson 1984; Leibenluft et al. 1987; C. A. Simpson and Porter 1981). Most commonly described is the use of cutting or taking handfuls of pills to convey anger or disappointment to the treater or other significant figures. Given the many reports that childhood abuse is common and discriminating for patients with BPD (Bryer et al. 1987; Herman et al. 1989; Links et al. 1988; Shearer et al. 1990; Stone 1981; Westen et al. 1990; Zanarini et al. 1989a), and given reports that their caretakers commonly fail to protect them or to validate their horrific experiences (see Chapter 3), it is understandable that borderline patients frequently resort to what has been described as a "hyperbolic stance," of which dramatic self-mutilation and suicide gestures may be seen as emblematic (Zanarini and Frankenburg 1994). This behavior may be understood as part of a greater effort to demand that attention be paid to the enormity of their pain (Zanarini and Frankenburg 1994).

Affect Dysregulation

It is well known that patients with BPD have great difficulty in experiencing and regulating affect (American Psychiatric

Association 1987; Gunderson 1984). It has been consistently reported that patients who inflict physical injury on themselves do so in an effort to terminate intensely dysphoric affects, often precipitated by real or perceived abandonment or neglect (Favazza 1989; Favazza and Conterio 1988, 1989; Gunderson 1984; Pattison and Kahan 1983; Rosenthal et al. 1972; M. A. Simpson 1977; C. A. Simpson and Porter 1981). There is evidence that early disruptions of attachment to primary caretakers through separation, abuse, or neglect may interfere with the development of biological systems of affective self-regulation (van der Kolk and Greenberg 1987). Researchers studying self-regulation in toddlers have been able to demonstrate this on a developmental-behavioral level. Cicchetti (1989) has reported that maltreated toddlers use fewer internal-state words and are less able to attribute internal states to social experiences than are nonmaltreated toddlers. He suggested that low tolerance for the expression of negative affect and inappropriate affective responsiveness by maltreating parents may prevent toddlers from being in touch with their feelings and may thereby lead to problems in the acquisition of emotional control.

In our sample of borderline subjects, inconsistent parental response, emotional withdrawal, and lack of protection by caregivers were characteristic childhood experiences of those who chronically self-mutilated. These conditions would make it especially difficult to develop the capacity to identify and label feelings, a necessary step in developing the capacity to make sense of and thereby manage feelings. In the face of traumatic experiences, self-protective mechanisms may develop, such as dissociation or depersonalization, psychic numbing, and physical analgesia (van der Kolk and Kadish 1987). Self-mutilation may then develop as both a way of self-stimulating (e.g., to feel real or alive again) and self-soothing (e.g., to alleviate overwhelming affects). Favazza (1989) described self-injurious behavior as a "purposeful if morbid act of self-help" (p. 143). In effect, these psychological processes and behaviors represent an adaptive, albeit pathological, form of affective regulation.

Biological Aspects

Several biological explanations for self-destructive behavior have been proposed in the literature. Van der Kolk and Greenberg (1987) suggested that this behavior may be related to possible trauma-induced psychophysiological changes involving an increase in neuronal excitability in the limbic system, leading to a kindling effect that interferes with normal mechanisms regulating affect and behavior. Findings from three studies by Teicher and colleagues, summarized in a recent report, supported this hypothesis (Teicher et al. 1994). These authors found both an increased prevalence of symptoms reflecting limbic system dysfunction and an increased prevalence of electroencephalographic (EEG) abnormalities in subjects who reported a history of childhood abuse. Using probe auditory-evoked potentials, they also found evidence to suggest that early trauma may affect the laterality of the developing brain, possibly leading to increased right-hemispheric activity or diminished hemispheric intercommunication. These investigators postulated that in individuals who suffer early traumatic experiences, greater reliance on the right hemisphere may contribute to the development of affective instability and impulsivity. This research suggests a role for trauma-induced neurodevelopmental abnormalities in the etiology of self-destructive behavior in some borderline patients. Dopaminergic systems have been implicated in the neurochemistry of self harm, and there is some evidence that dysregulation of opiate systems may be involved, including several case reports of positive effects of opiate antagonists in diminishing self-destructive behavior (Winchel et al. 1991). There is also recent research suggesting that underlying serotonergic dysfunction may facilitate suicidal behavior and self-mutilation (Simeon et al. 1992; Winchel and Stanley 1991).

Despite recent advances in the biological understanding of self-destructive behavior, empirical evidence for the efficacy of medications in treating self-destructive behavior in patients with BPD has been limited. Most reports of the pharmacological treatment of borderline patients have not addressed specific effects on self-injurious behavior. Gardner and Cowdry (1985, 1986) carried out a multidrug double-blind crossover study comparing

the effects of trifluoperazine, alprazolam, tranylcypromine, carbamazepine, and placebo on specific borderline symptoms,
including self-destructive behavior. Only treatment with carbamazepine resulted in a significant decrease in self-destructive episodes.

Treatment Implications

In the only study to date comparing the effectiveness of cognitive-
behavioral treatment with that of other forms of psychotherapy in chronically self-destructive borderline patients,
cognitive-behavior therapy had a better outcome (Linehan et al.
1991, 1993). The treatment developed by Linehan focused on
developing more effective coping strategies by building skills in
emotion regulation, distress tolerance, interpersonal effectiveness, and self-management. Validation of the patient's experiences and feelings and communication of nonjudgmental
understanding of the patient's behavior were emphasized (Linehan 1987).

Authors writing about childhood trauma and BPD have also
emphasized the importance of emotional validation of the borderline patient's experiences and benevolent understanding of
their behavior for success in treatment. These psychotherapeutic
approaches are first steps in helping patients with BPD to identify and label their feelings, thereby increasing their capacity for
self-reflection and control over self-destructive impulses (Perry
et al. 1990; Zanarini and Frankenburg 1994). It is possible that
psychodynamic psychotherapy did not fare well in the study by
Linehan (1987) because of the frequent problem of emphasis on
the meaning of self-destructive acts without the incorporation of
concrete cognitive-behavioral approaches to help manage the
behavior. Another common problem is lack of agreed-on contingency planning for suicidal behavior, which would include
a continuum from self-soothing behaviors through hospitalization (Kernberg 1989). Without such an understanding with
the patient, struggles are more apt to arise around whether the
therapist cares enough (e.g., to be available for frequent phone
calls at all hours or for extended sessions), and the treatment
becomes a test of the therapist's capacity to "save" the patient.
Disappointment and anger by both patient and therapist are

likely to ensue, which usually exacerbates the patient's self-destructive behavior (Gunderson 1984; Kernberg et al. 1989). It would seem that an integrative approach to treatment is most efficacious. This would involve validation of the patient's feelings and experiences, empathic understanding of the purpose self-harm serves for the patient in regulating affect and communicating distress, linking present-day triggers of affect intolerance with past traumas, and establishing more adaptive strategies for managing overwhelming feelings, all within a therapeutic structure in which maintaining safety is a mutually-agreed-on treatment goal.

CONCLUSIONS

By assessing lifetime patterns of self-harm, our study revealed three significant findings related to the phenomenology of this behavior in borderline patients. Our results confirmed previous reports that chronic, repetitive self-destructive behavior discriminates borderline patients from other patient groups, even very near neighbors. We also identified a subgroup of patients who reported childhood onset of self-harm; and we described a subgroup of super self-destructive borderline subjects, who accounted for nearly half our sample. Differences between subgroups are probably multifactorial, reflecting constitutional, psychological, and early environmental influences. Most important, our findings provided further confirmation of the strong association between chronic self-destructive behavior and childhood histories of both parental sexual abuse and emotional neglect in patients with BPD. Awareness of the role of childhood abuse and neglect in the etiology of self-destructive behavior in borderline patients can help treaters to be more empathic and to have greater understanding of borderline patients' desperate, ill-fated attempts to manage their feelings and experiences. With this nonjudgmental perspective, the therapist can engage the patient in linking present-day feelings and reactions to past trauma and deprivation and in developing more adaptive mechanisms of self-regulation.

REFERENCES

American Psychiatric Association: Diagnostic and Statistical Manual of Mental Disorders, 3rd Edition, Revised. Washington, DC, American Psychiatric Press, 1987

Andrulonis PA, Glueck BC, Stroebel CF, et al: Organic brain dysfunction and the borderline syndrome. Psychiatr Clin North Am 4:47–66, 1981

Bach-y-Rita G: Habitual violence and self-mutilation. Am J Psychiatry 131:1018–1020, 1974

Barrash J, Kroll J, Carey K, et al: Discriminating BPD from other personality disorders: cluster analyses of the Diagnostic Interview for Borderlines. Arch Gen Psychiatry 40:1297–1302, 1983

Browne A, Finkelhor D: Impact of child sexual abuse: a review of the research. Psychol Bull 99:66–77, 1986

Bryer JB, Nelson BA, Miller JB, et al: Childhood sexual and physical abuse as factors in adult psychiatric illness. Am J Psychiatry 144:1426–1430, 1987

Carroll J, Schaffer C, Spensley J, et al: Family experiences of self-mutilating patients. Am J Psychiatry 137:852–853, 1980

Cicchetti D: How research on child maltreatment has informed the study of child development: perspectives from developmental psychology, in Child Maltreatment. Edited by Cicchetti D, Carlson V. Cambridge, England, Cambridge University Press, 1989, pp 377–431

de Wilde EJ, Kienhorst CW, Diekstra RF, et al: The relationship between adolescent suicidal behavior and life events in childhood and adolescence. Am J Psychiatry 149:45–51, 1992

Dulit RA, Fyer MR, Leon AC, et al: Clinical correlates of self-mutilation in borderline personality disorder. Am J Psychiatry 151:1305–1311, 1994

Favazza AR: Why patients mutilate themselves. Hosp Community Psychiatry 40:137–145, 1989

Favazza AR, Conterio K: The plight of chronic self-mutilators. Community Ment Health J 24:22–30, 1988

Favazza AR, Conterio K: Female habitual self-mutilators. Acta Psychiatr Scand 79:283–289, 1989

Frances A: Introduction. J Personality Disorders 1:316, 1987

Frances A, Clarkin JF, Gilmore M, et al: Reliability of criteria for BPD: a comparison of DSM-III and the Diagnostic Interview for Borderline Patients. Am J Psychiatry 141:1080–1084, 1984

Gardner DL, Cowdry RW: Suicidal and parasuicidal behavior in BPD. Psychiatr Clin North Am 8:389–403, 1985

Gardner DL, Cowdry RW: Positive effects of carbamazepine on behavioral dyscontrol in BPD. Am J Psychiatry 143:519–522, 1986

Green A: Self-destructive behavior in battered children. Am J Psychiatry 135:579–582, 1978

Grunebaum HU, Klerman GL: Wrist slashing. Am J Psychiatry 124:527–534, 1967

Gunderson JG: Borderline Personality Disorder. Washington, DC, American Psychiatric Press, 1984

Gunderson JG, Zanarini MC: Pathogenesis of borderline personality, in The American Psychiatric Press Review of Psychiatry, Vol 8. Edited by Frances AJ, Hales RE, Tasman A. Washington, DC: American Psychiatric Press, 1989, pp 25–48

Gunderson JG, Kolb JE, Austin V: The Diagnostic Interview for Borderline Patients. Am J Psychiatry 138: 896–903, 1981

Herman JL, Perry JC, van der Kolk BA: Childhood trauma in BPD. Am J Psychiatry 146:490–495, 1989

Kernberg OF, Selzer MA, Koenigsberg HW, et al: Psychodynamic Psychotherapy of Borderline Patients. New York, Basic Books, 1989

Leibenluft E, Gardner DL, Cowdry RW: The inner experience of the borderline self-mutilator. Journal of Personality Disorders 1:317–324, 1987

Linehan M: Dialectical Behavioral Therapy: a cognitive behavioral approach to parasuicide. Journal of Personality Disorders 1:328–333, 1987

Linehan M, Armstrong HE, Suarez A, et al: Cognitive-behavioral treatment of chronically parasuicidal borderline patients. Arch Gen Psychiatry 48:1060–1064, 1991

Linehan M, Heard H, Armstrong HE: Naturalistic follow-up of a behavioral treatment for chronically parasuicidal borderline patients. Arch Gen Psychiatry 50:971–974, 1993

Links PS, Steiner M, Offord DR, et al: Characteristics of BPD: a Canadian study. Can J Psychiatry 33:336–340, 1988

Links PS, Boiago I, Huxley G, et al: Sexual abuse and biparental failure as etiologic models in BPD, in Family Environment and Borderline Personality Disorder. Edited by Links PS. American Psychiatric Press, Washington, DC, 1990, pp 107–120

Pattison EM, Kahan J: The deliberate self-harm syndrome. Am J Psychiatry 140:867–872, 1983

Perry JC: Personality disorders, suicide, and self-destructive behavior, in Suicide: Understanding and Responding: Harvard Medical School Perspectives. Edited by Jacobs D, Brown H. Madison, CT, International Universities Press, 1989, pp 157–169

Perry JC, Herman JL, van der Kolk BA, et al: Psychotherapy and psychological trauma in BPD. Psychiatric Annals 20:33–43, 1990

Rosenthal PA, Rosenthal S: Suicidal behavior by preschool children. Am J Psychiatry 141:520–524, 1984

Rosenthal RJ, Rinzler C, Wallsh R, et al: Wrist cutting syndrome: the meaning of a gesture. Am J Psychiatry 128:1363–1368, 1972

Roy A: Self-mutilation. Br J Med Psychol 51:201–203, 1978

Russ MJ, Shearin EN, Clarkin JF, et al: Subtypes of self-injurious patients with BPD. Am J Psychiatry 150:1869–1871, 1993

Schaffer CB, Carroll J, Abramowitz SI: Self-mutilation and the borderline personality. J Nerv Ment Dis 170:468–473, 1982

Shearer SL, Peters CP, Quaytman MS, et al: Intent and lethality of suicide attempts among female borderline inpatients. Am J Psychiatry 145:1424–1427, 1988

Shearer SL, Peters CP, Quaytman MS, et al: Frequency and correlates of childhood sexual and physical abuse histories in adult female borderline inpatients. Am J Psychiatry 147:214–216, 1990

Simeon D, Stanley B, Frances A, et al: Self-mutilation in personality disorders: psychological and biological correlates. Am J Psychiatry 149:221–226, 1992

Simpson CA, Porter GL: Self-mutilation in children and adolescents. Bull Menninger Clin 45:428–438, 1981

Simpson MA: Self-mutilation and the borderline syndrome. Dynamische Psychiatrie 10:42–48, 1977

Soloff PH, Lis JA, Kelly T, et al: Risk factors for suicidal behavior in BPD. Am J Psychiatry 151:1316–1323, 1994

Stone MH: Borderline syndromes: a consideration of subtypes and an overview, directions for research. Psychiatr Clin North Am 4:3–23, 1981

Stone MH: A psychodynamic approach: some thoughts on the dynamics and therapy of self-mutilating borderline patients. Journal of Personality Disorders 1:347–349, 1987

Teicher MH, Ito Y, Glod CA, et al: Early abuse, limbic system dysfunction, and BPD, in Biological and Neurobehavioral Studies of Borderline Personality Disorder. Edited by Silk KR. Washington, DC, American Psychiatric Press, 1994, pp 177–207

van der Kolk BA, Greenberg MS: The psychobiology of the trauma response: hyperarousal, constriction, and addiction to traumatic reexposure, in Psychological Trauma. Edited by van der Kolk BA. Washington, DC, American Psychiatric Press, 1987, pp 63–87

van der Kolk BA, Kadish W: Amnesia, dissociation, and the return of the repressed, in Psychological Trauma. Edited by van der Kolk BA. Washington, DC, American Psychiatric Press, 1987, pp 173–190

van der Kolk BA, Perry JC, Herman JL: Childhood origins of self-destructive behavior. Am J Psychiatry 148:1665–1671, 1991

Westen D, Ludolph P, Misle B, et al: Physical and sexual abuse in adolescent girls with BPD. Am J Orthopsychiatry 60:55–66, 1990

Winchel RM, Stanley M: Self-injurious behavior: a review of the behavior and biology of self-mutilation. Am J Psychiatry 148:306–317, 1991

Zanarini MC, Frankenburg FR: Emotional hypochondriasis, hyperbole, and the borderline patient. Journal of Psychotherapy Practice and Research 3:25–36, 1994

Zanarini MC, Gunderson JG, Marino MF, et al: Childhood experiences of borderline patients. Compr Psychiatry 30:18–25, 1989a

Zanarini MC, Gunderson JG, Frankenburg FR, et al: The Revised Diagnostic Interview for Borderlines: discriminating BPD from other Axis II disorders. J Personality Disorders 3:10–18, 1989b

Zanarini MC, Gunderson JG, Frankenburg FR, et al: Discriminating BPD from other Axis II disorders. Am J Psychiatry 147:161–167, 1990

Chapter 8

Severity of Childhood Sexual Abuse, Borderline Symptoms, and Familial Environment

Kenneth R. Silk, M.D., Joel T. Nigg, Ph.D.,
Drew Westen, Ph.D., and Naomi E. Lohr, Ph.D.

In 1981 Michael Stone made the following prescient observation:

> I suspect there is another and purely psychogenic factor contributing to the excess of females among groups of borderline patients. . . . the occurrence of incestuous experiences during childhood or adolescence. . . . Brooks has recently been collecting data on a population of hospitalized borderline patients; although the sample is still small (12 women with a diagnosis of borderline by Kernberg's [Kernberg 1975] criteria), the incidence of incest was strikingly high—75%. . . . Chronic victimization of this sort, by a father or an uncle, cannot help but have damaging effects upon the psychic development of a young girl. These effects will generally consist of impaired relationships with men, mistrust of men, inordinate preoccupation with sexual themes, impulsivity in the area of sex, and often enough, depression. . . . Perceptions of self and others . . . are overdrawn and contradictory. (pp. 14–15)

The publication of this book attests to the recent increase in empirical research in the relationship between borderline personality disorder (BPD) and antecedent sexual and/or physical abuse. We discuss the approach we have taken in the Personality Disorders Program in the Department of Psychiatry at the University of Michigan Medical Center, and we present the results from our studies. Our ongoing research into the relationship between sexual abuse and BPD began in 1987.

VERACITY OF RETROSPECTIVE
SEXUAL ABUSE DATA

The use of retrospective data requires proper framing in psychopathology research, but recent attention in the literature and in the media to possible false reports of abuse (termed *false memory syndromes* by advocates) compels that research reports such as ours be placed explicitly in the appropriate perspective. We therefore deemed it important in writing this chapter to give serious consideration to the veracity of retrospective reports.

Historically, society as well as clinical theory and practice have undergone periodic enlightenment and retrenchment in regard to the evidence that sexual abuse is a serious social problem (Olafson et al. 1993). The publication of some 30 studies since the mid-1980s documenting the frequency, severity, and sequelae of sexual abuse (Kendall-Tackett et al. 1993) has been accompanied, as in the past, by controversy over false memories (Dittburner and Persinger 1993; Frankel 1993; Grinfeld and Reisman 1993; Gross 1994) as well as by sympathy for allegedly falsely accused perpetrators and claims that sexual abuse is overblown as a societal problem (e.g., Gardner 1991). Allegations of false reports tend to emphasize case examples of questionable clinical practice (e.g., use of drugs to aid "recall") and target reports of bizarre and ritualistic abuse (e.g., Ofshe 1992; Ofshe and Waters 1993). Indeed, memory can be influenced by suggestion and can even be implanted in the laboratory under certain conditions (Loftus 1993). However, such data are of dubious etiological validity regarding the impact of trauma on development and on memory and are not informed by clinical practice or clinical theory. As a result, the contribution of the false memory debate to clinical theory/practice and to psychopathology research is not yet apparent.

In particular, demonstration that sexual abuse memories can be implanted has not been provided. By contrast, when suggestion is not an issue, the data, on balance, support the veracity of memories for autobiographical events, including trauma, despite the accepted unreliability of specific details in nearly all human memory (Brewin et al. 1993).

However, these critiques raise another underexplored issue: if some patients are suggestible for memories of trauma, why are they so suggestible? The literature on hypnosis and personality suggests that a history of trauma may predispose adults to fantasy proneness and suggestibility (Lynn and Rhue 1988). Ironically, then, suggestibility for traumatic memories may be one more symptom of trauma, along with dissociation and related sequelae. Exploration of this issue will be crucial to clarifying the clinical issues related to treatment of trauma victims. It is to be hoped that future research will move beyond premature certainty to address such complexities empirically.

As is generally acknowledged, both controlled studies of repression and controlled, prospective longitudinal studies of the impact of trauma on development are lacking. This fact requires researchers to suspend final judgment on models of psychopathology that depend on retrospective recall. But our scientific responsibility does not end there. Rather, some estimate of the validity of retrospective reports of abuse is crucial.

As noted, apart from the issue of recovery of repressed memories (discussed later), the evidence to date suggests that retrospective reports by psychiatric patients are generally as accurate as any other retrospective reports (Brewin et al. 1993). Depression is sometimes thought to bias recall negatively (Lewinsohn and Rosenbaum 1987), although on balance the evidence seems to suggest that depressed individuals' memories are reliable (Brewin et al. 1993). Because depressed mood is one feature of BPD, our use of a severely depressed non-BPD comparison group in our research ensures that findings are not due to depressed mood.

The role of repression in recall deserves further mention. In the limited empirical examination of various theories of repression, it appears that repression can occur around specific affectively charged and threatening memories (Davis 1987). The reality of some form of amnesia (whether repression or some other process) for trauma, in turn, has been shown by Williams (1992), who followed 100 women who had been sexually abused as children (abuse was documented from hospital emergency room reports when the women were children). Of these women, 38 had no memory of the trauma, even under leading questioning. Herman and Schatzow (1987) found that the majority of patients who recovered memories in group therapy could objectively verify those memories later. An earlier report by us (Nigg et al. 1991) showed verification of a majority of abuse reports, and Briere and Conte (1993) found that among 450 adult psychiatric patients who reported a history of abuse, 59% reported a period when they were unable to recall the abuse experiences. Hence, possible underreporting of abuse is apparently a more serious obstacle to accurate retrospective research than is overreporting.

Our data collection began in 1987, before the recent media attention to these questions. Hence it is unlikely that our subjects were influenced by media reports linking abuse to psychiatric problems. In our own data we have made further efforts to examine the credibility of memories, qualitatively and empirically.

Qualitatively, several considerations are pertinent. First, our information comes from an observer-rated structured interview. Second, the abuse questions are embedded in a much longer interview (questions 19–25 out of 40), so that propensity to yea-saying would be unlikely to occur only for one portion (e.g., the sexual abuse portion) of the interview. At the same time, some rapport had occurred by this point in the interview. Third, the interview was administered by clinicians and not lay interviewers, and clinicians are more likely to evaluate response veracity in the light of responses to the remainder of the interview.

Further, one clue to veracity is that fictitious accounts, at least in children, are accompanied by particular clinical features such as lack of emotion (Jones and McGraw 1987); in adults, one would assume that emphasis would be placed on oneself being victimized if a false recollection were psychologically motivated. Yet, as many of our subjects later discussed in their treatment, the idea of having been sexually abused as a child often meant that they themselves, and not their abusers, were the bad persons. They (the abused) must have done something wrong, or must have wanted the abuse to happen, or must have been seductive. There was (and remains) among most of our patients, very little propensity to blame the abuser. Further, when subjects reported abuse, their affect and demeanor were almost always consistent with their discussing a seriously disturbing aspect of their childhood. Subjects often revealed shame, embarrassment, and reluctance in discussing the abuse.

Empirically, we interviewed informants (usually mothers) independently in 20 cases (selected blind to abuse report). Parents tend to provide more optimistic recollections of their children's lives than do the children (Brewin et al. 1993); hence, parental reports of abuse are unlikely to be fabricated. Of these 20, 11 were informants for subjects who had reported abuse. Of those 11 informants, 8 independently confirmed the sexual abuse history. Of the 9 informants for patients (subjects) who had not reported abuse, 3 stated that the subject had been sexually abused as a child. These data suggest, if one believes the disagreements are of equal validity, that underreporting is equal in magnitude to overreporting but that both occur in a minority of cases. Given the propensity of parents to underreport, it is more likely that our data from patients are characterized by slight underreporting of abuse than by overreporting. However, the rates of abuse reported by subjects in our studies are quite consistent with those in other research centers with various comparison groups (Herman et al. 1989; Westen et al. 1990b; Zanarini et al. 1989); it would be surprising if the same percentage of fabricated reports occurred across several research sites. On balance, then, it appears most parsimonious to view the retrospective reports as largely accurate regarding the main features of presence or absence, and probably severity, of abuse. As many of the papers in this volume suggest, borderline patients have experienced more severe sexual abuse than have comparison groups.

SEXUAL ABUSE SEQUELAE, OBJECT RELATIONS, AND MALEVOLENCE

The initial effects of sexual abuse include fear, anxiety, depression, guilt, anger, hostility, and inappropriate sexual behavior (Briere and Runtz 1986; Browne and Finkelhor 1986; Herman et al. 1986; Jason et al. 1982; Sedney and Brooks 1984). The long-term sequelae include impulsivity, self-blame, suicidal behavior, anxiety, feelings of isolation, poor self-esteem, substance abuse, sexual problems, lack of interpersonal trust, depression, and self-mutilation (Browne and Finkelhor 1986; Carmen et al. 1984; Green 1983; Herman et al. 1986; A. Jacobson and Richardson

1987; Russell 1984). These long-term sequelae overlap with many of the symptoms often seen in borderline patients, and in 1987, Herman and van der Kolk postulated that some BPD patients, and perhaps the majority of female BPD patients, were suffering from posttraumatic stress disorder. Using this approach, many of the symptoms of BPD could also, and perhaps, more correctly, be viewed as the result of early childhood trauma, particularly sexual abuse (Gunderson and Sabo 1993).

We have long been interested in the clinical and interpersonal manifestations of object relations of borderline patients (Westen et al. 1990a). We have been particularly interested in trying to understand better the borderline patient's expectation of encountering a malevolent world (Westen 1990). This expectation of malevolence has been noticed by others, who have speculated about its possible origins as well as its development in transference during psychotherapy with the borderline patient (Kernberg 1975; Masterson 1976).

In this chapter we review four studies conducted at the University of Michigan between 1987 and 1993. The first study looked at which BPD symptoms are most predictive of sexual abuse. The second study explored the early memories of BPD patients with respect to memories of deliberate injury and the depiction of severely malevolent characters in those memories. The third and fourth studies explored dimensions of the severity of sexual abuse among abused borderline patients and abused non-BPD control groups. The third study examined which parameters of severity of sexual abuse experiences predicted specific symptoms of BPD, as defined by the Diagnostic Interview for Borderlines (DIB) (Gunderson et al. 1981); and the last study explored the influence of diagnosis and of the severity of abuse on the recalled family environments of abused versus nonabused subjects.

GENERAL METHODOLOGY

Subjects

Subjects for whom BPD and major depressive disorder were diagnosed were recruited from two inpatient psychiatry units at the University of Michigan Medical Center. Male and female inpatients ages 18–60 who fulfilled at least two DSM-III-R criteria (American Psychiatric Association 1987) for BPD or schizotypal personality disorder, or three criteria for major depressive episode, were considered potential subjects. Factors excluding patients from consideration were organicity, chronic psychosis, or a native language other than English.

Eighty-five percent of potential subjects agreed to participate in the research. Diagnosis of borderline was made with the DIB by a research team member. Our group's reliability (kappa = .8) for the DIB has been established (Cornell et al. 1983) and maintained through periodic retraining. Patients who scored ≥ 7 on the DIB were included in the borderline cohort. Patients who scored ≤ 5 on the DIB and who also met Research Diagnostic Criteria (RDC) (Spitzer et al. 1975) for major depressive disorder (MDD) were the nonborderline depressed control subjects. Senior supervisors who were research group members and who had obtained good interrater reliability for the diagnosis of major depressive disorder (weighted kappa = .92) made the RDC diagnoses. Both supervisor and therapist were blind to DIB results. Subjects scoring 6 on the DIB were intentionally excluded in advance to minimize group overlap. We had initially chosen a depressed control group in order to explore the interface between BPD and MDD (Gold and Silk 1993; Gunderson and Phillips 1991). However, in sexual abuse research, chronic depression is often seen as a long-term result of sexual abuse. Therefore, the selection of this control group seemed particularly useful for this aspect of our research.

Psychiatrically healthy subjects were recruited through public advertisements requesting volunteers "in good physical and emotional health who have never been in psychotherapy and are reasonably content with their lives." All potential psychiatrically healthy control subjects were given the Minnesota Multiphasic Personality Inventory (MMPI) (Hathaway and McKinley 1989) as well as the Rosenberg Self-Esteem Scale (Rosenberg 1965). Our recruitment of psychiatrically healthy subjects is explained in detail elsewhere (Benjamin et al. 1989; Nigg et al. 1992).

A total of 89 subjects were recruited in this manner over a number of years. The studies reported here have different numbers of subjects because the research has been ongoing, and different studies have been conducted at different stages in the process. Within this total cohort, 55 met DIB criteria for BPD, 18 met RDC criteria for MDD without meeting DIB criteria for BPD, 15 met our screening for psychiatrically healthy control subjects, and 1 met criteria for a different psychiatric disorder (anxiety disorder). Of this total cohort, 51 reported sexual abuse on the Familial Experience Interview (FEI) (see below): 41 from the borderline group, 7 from the depressed control subjects, and 3 from the normal control subjects.

Familial Experiences Interview

Members of the research team who were blind to both the DIB and the RDC results interviewed all subjects with the FEI (Ogata et al. 1990b). The FEI was developed by Ogata in collaboration with members of our research team. The interview explores a variety of early childhood/familial events, including loss, separation, illness, school problems, abuse (physical and sexual), and neglect (Ogata 1989). Questions were in the same sequence for all subjects. *Sexual abuse* was broadly defined along a continuum, from exposure to genitals with no physical contact, through fondling or caressing of genitals, to penetration. Only 1 case of our 51 cases was exposure. Specific questions were asked about sexual activity between subject and father, mother, siblings, relatives (assessed for biological as well as nonbiological relatives), and people outside the family. Each question was also scored for frequency (did not occur, discrete episodes, ongoing), severity (exposure without contact, fondling or caressing, penetration), duration (up to 1 year, 1–5 years, longer than 5 years), and emotional impact. Weighted kappas for all but 6 of the 150 total items on the FEI were above .70. No item used in any analysis discussed in this chapter had a weighted kappa below .70 (Ogata 1989). These procedures apply to each of the studies described below.

STUDY 1: BPD SYMPTOMS AND SEXUAL ABUSE

Study 1 explored these questions: Had borderline patients experienced a greater incidence of physical, sexual, or both physical and sexual abuse during childhood than depressed patients, and if so, in what ways? Were particular BPD symptoms, as measured by the DIB, more likely to predict the past occurrence of sexual abuse?

We formed three hypotheses: 1) More borderline than non-borderline patients would report sexual and physical abuse histories. 2) Sexual abuse would predict the BPD diagnosis. 3) Predictors of sexual abuse would be found among DIB items relating to impulsivity, dissociative experiences, and disordered personal relationships—areas within which, on the DIB, the long-term consequences of abuse (as reported in the literature and summarized above) might be found.

Results

There were 24 BPD patients and 18 depressed control subjects in this sample; 71% (17) of the borderline patients, compared to 22% (4) of the depressed control subjects, reported a history of childhood sexual abuse ($\chi^2 = 7.88$, df = 1, $P = .005$). Although 42% (10/24) of the borderline subjects reported physical abuse, this was not a statistically significant difference from the 33% (6/18) of the depressed control subjects who also reported physical abuse. Only 17% (4/24) of the borderline subjects and 6% (1/18) of the depressed control subjects reported physical neglect. Thus the first hypothesis was partially supported. BPD subjects had significantly greater reported frequency of sexual but not physical abuse than did depressed patients.

A stepwise logistic regression was performed with diagnosis as the dependent variable and six abuse variables as predictors: any sexual abuse, any physical abuse, any physical neglect, sexual abuse perpetrated by a nuclear family member, sexual abuse perpetrated by other relatives, and sexual abuse perpetrated by nonrelatives. This was done to examine whether a specific type of abuse might predict the diagnosis of BPD. Sexual abuse was the only significant predictor when all variables were forced to be tested in the model until the residual variance was nonsignificant, both when all the subjects were included ($\chi^2 = 10.18$, df = 1, $P = .0014$) and when the sample was restricted to only women ($\chi^2 = 9.72$, df = 1, $P = .0018$) (because only 1 man reported sexual abuse). Thus the second hypothesis, that sexual abuse (when comparing borderline patients with depressed patients) significantly predicts the BPD diagnosis, was supported (Ogata et al. 1990b).

To test the third hypothesis, a second series of stepwise logistic regressions were run to determine whether certain DIB items could predict sexual abuse. We chose five individual DIB items as predictor variables: promiscuity, chronic dysphoria (as manifested by emptiness, loneliness, and boredom), derealization, depersonalization, and dependent and/or masochistic relationships. These DIB items are frequently mentioned in the psychiatric literature as adult sequelae of childhood sexual abuse. Two additional predictors were created and entered: 1) a symptom predictor that consisted of the remaining DIB items (not counted among the five above) that related to social presentation, affective functioning, and transient psychosis and 2) an interpersonal relationship predictor that consisted of the DIB items remaining in the interpersonal relationship and impulsivity sections after removing all previously mentioned items. The predictor values were derived by summing the positive responses on the respective DIB items that made up each predictor.

When all subjects were included in the regression, significant predictors were derealization and promiscuity ($\chi^2 = 25.98$, df = 1, $P < .0001$). However, everyone who was promiscuous also acknowledged experiencing derealization, and thus promiscuity did not remain a significant predictor after derealization was in the model. When the analysis was restricted to only female subjects, chronic dysphoria marked by emptiness, loneliness, and boredom was the only significant predictor of sexual abuse ($\chi^2 = 8.89$, df = 1, $P < .005$). Thus our third hypothesis was only partially supported. There were specific DIB items that could predict the reported presence of childhood sexual abuse, but these predictors were not from the impulsivity or the personal relationship sections of the DIB. However, they did relate to dissociation, which is found in the psychosis subsection of the DIB. Promiscuity is found in the impulse subsection, and chronic dysphoria is found in the affect subsection of the DIB. Thus, no particular subsection of the DIB was correlated to a history of sexual abuse.

STUDY 2: EARLY MEMORIES, SEXUAL ABUSE, AND MALEVOLENT OBJECT REPRESENTATIONS

We then examined more closely how the experience of sexual abuse might manifest itself in the borderline patients' object relations, that is, in their self and other representations. We were interested in what kinds of interpersonal expectations BPD patients and victims of childhood sexual abuse had and what kinds of assumptions they made. According to psychoanalytic theory, borderline patients suffer from pathological object relations (Kernberg 1976). Internal ideational representations of others and the self, as well as the expectations and affects attached to them, are what is usually defined as object representations (E. Jacobson 1964; Nigg et al. 1992; Sandler and Rosenblatt 1961).

To provide a measure of the object representations or inner relationship schema, we administered the Early Memories Test to patients (Bruhn and Last 1982; Mayman 1968; Mayman and Faris 1960; Taylor 1975). The Early Memories Test consists of open-ended probes of the subject—for example, "Tell me your earliest memory." The Early Memories Test was considered a projective test; that is, it is assumed that the subject undergoes some internal process of selection and filtering, as well as reconstruction, in responding to the prompt (Bruhn and Last 1982; Exner 1993).

The responses related by the subjects thus reflect their personality, what is salient to them, and hence their mental representations of their interpersonal world and the affective meanings attached (termed *the inner object world*). The responses to this task are hence quite different in meaning from responses to probes in the structured interview about family experiences (FEI), which asks specifically about particular events and hence does not allow the subjects total freedom to select their recollections. We hypothesized that sexually abused subjects, regardless of diagnosis, would more frequently report memories in which some injury occurred (reflecting the salience of abuse in their mental representations). Further, we hypothesized that in these narratives, others would be portrayed as more malevolent, and potential helpers as less helpful, than in the narratives of comparison subjects, including those with major depression.

Methods

The general subject selection method was as explained earlier. As part of a battery of psychological tests, all subjects were given a modified version of Mayman's Early Memories Test (Mayman 1968; Mayman and Faris 1960). Subjects were asked to relate 12 specific early memories, but in the current analysis we used only 4 memories. We used the earliest, the next earliest, the earliest of mother, and the earliest of father memories, because these questions are affectively neutral; hence they are most likely to allow expression of individual variation in affect tone of their responses. Typed verbatim transcripts of the memories were sorted by type of memory to prevent rater halo effect among all the memories of a particular subject. Two coders rated each transcript, and discrepancies were resolved by consensus.

Scoring was done as follows: deliberate injury was defined as present when the memory included intentional attack or assault with physical contact, and it could include pushing, shoving, or hitting. If no physical contact or injury occurred, then deliberate injury was not scored even if the threat of physical or emotional harm was present. If the memory included a sexual assault, the sexual assault was not counted as injury to avoid confounding dependent and independent variables, although other injuries in those memories would be counted. Injuries were scored as yes or no (kappa = .95). Helper effectiveness was scored on a 5-point ordinal type of scale (.83 weighted kappa) as follows: 1 = no helper present, 2 = helper present but made no attempt to help or was oblivious to the problem, 3 = helper attempted to intervene but was ineffective, 4 = helper provided partial relief, comfort, or protection, and 5 = helper provided complete relief, recovery, or protection. Affect tone was scored on a 5-point continuous scale developed by Barends et al. (1990) (uncorrected intraclass correlation coefficient = .78, Spearman-Brown correction = .88). This scale measured "the affective quality of representations of people and relationships, or interpersonal expectancies portrayed, from malevolent to benevolent" (Nigg et al. 1991, p. 866): 1 = unambivalently malevolent or destructive, 2 = hostile, empty, but not profoundly malevolent and not a threat to one's existence, 3 = mixed, with a mild negative tone but capable of caring,

4 = mixed, with a neutral to positive tone, with people generally depicted as caring for and enjoying one another, and 5 = predominantly positive, kind, warm, where intimacy, love, and loyalty can be expected.

Results

Of the 58 subjects in this study, 29 were diagnosed with BPD, 14 were diagnosed with major depression without BPD, and 15 were screened psychiatrically healthy control subjects. Seventy-two percent (21/29) of the borderline subjects, 29% (4/14) of the depressed subjects, and 20% (3/15) of the psychiatrically healthy control subjects reported sexual abuse in childhood ($\chi^2 = 13.8$, df = 2, $P < .01$). Forty-eight percent (28/58) of the entire sample reported sexual abuse during childhood.

Early Memories Test responses of deliberate injury were significantly more frequent among the sexually abused subjects (11/28) than among the subjects not sexually abused (0/30) (Fisher's exact $P = .0001$). Among the borderline patients as well, 9 of the 21 abused subjects recalled memories in which deliberate injury took place, whereas none of the 8 nonabused borderline patients recalled memories with deliberate injury (Fisher's exact $P = .03$). In fact, only subjects who were sexually abused reported memories that were coded positive for deliberate injury.

A logistic regression was performed to test for possible confounding data. When age was controlled for, sexual abuse was a significant predictor of injury in the early memories ($\chi^2 = 12.1$, df = 1, $P = .0005$), whereas physical abuse ($\chi^2 = 1.71$, df = 1) and diagnosis ($\chi^2 = 2.68$, df = 2) were not significant. Thus, sexually abused subjects clearly had more deliberate injuries in their early memories, and because 75% of the abused subjects were borderline patients, borderline patients had the majority of the memories containing deliberate injury. Of the 11 subjects who reported memories with deliberate injury, 9 were borderline subjects and 2 were depressed, but none were among the 3 abused psychiatrically healthy control subjects. Fifty-seven percent (33) of the subjects received the Early Memories Test before receiving the FEI. Order of administration was unrelated to frequency of Early Memories Test injury responses (χ^2 = .07, df = 1, NS).

There was no relationship between effectiveness of helpers and abuse when all four types of memories were combined. However, in the earliest memories of mother, mothers in the memories of the nonabused subjects were seen as significantly more helpful than mothers in the memories of the abused subjects (t = 2.33, df = 9, P = .04). Thus our second hypothesis, that abused subjects' memories would depict less helpful people, was partially supported.

Of interest is that when all subjects were considered, abused subjects' memories received significantly lower (i.e., more malevolent) scores for affect tone than did nonabused subjects' memories (abused = 2.76 versus nonabused = 3.27: t = 2.75, df = 54, P = .01). However, when only borderline patients were considered, although the abused borderline subjects' affect tone was lower (2.55) than the nonabused borderline subjects' affect tone (3.00), the difference was not significant (t = 1.29, df = 26). Only sexually abused BPD subjects gave Early Memories Test responses that depicted characters in the most malevolent category. Thus the responses of abused subjects contained both much more negative affect tone and more frequent extremely malevolent character depictions than did the responses of nonabused subjects. A logistic regression found that sexual abuse rather than diagnosis or physical abuse was a significant predictor of malevolent character depictions (χ^2 = 5.19, df = 1, P < .03), and a multiple regression found that sexual abuse was a predictor of negative affect tone (t = –2.46, df = 47, P = .02) and that BPD diagnosis revealed a trend toward the prediction of negative affect in the memories (F = 3.00, df = 2,46, P = .06). When both sexual abuse and diagnosis were tested simultaneously, neither provided significant additional information over the other (Nigg et al. 1991).

This second study suggested that sexual abuse and borderline personality are both predictive of malevolent expectations of personal relationships. This finding would be consistent with the idea that sexual abuse is one but not the only pathway to the development of such malevolent interpersonal schemas. Further, patients with a diagnosis of BPD who report a history of sexual abuse are particularly likely to experience malevolent expectations of others. Along with this result, helpers may be experienced as unhelpful, an expectation pertinent to clinical intervention strategies (Nigg et al. 1992).

STUDY 3: SEVERITY OF SEXUAL ABUSE AND BPD SYMPTOMS

Not all subjects who reported sexual abuse had Early Memories Test responses in which injury was depicted, and not all subjects who were abused depicted malevolent characters in their memories. We hypothesized that the type (specific act or specific perpetrator) and the frequency of the sexual abuse might account for why some people survive sexual abuse with few psychopathological sequelae and others develop serious psychopathology.

Although borderline patients are not the only people or patients who have been abused, in the majority of cases the sexual abuse alleged among borderline patients is not a single event or an event with a stranger (Silk et al. 1993). (See Paris and Zweig-Frank, Chapter 2, this volume, for a different set of results pertaining to the parameters of sexual abuse among a sample of borderline outpatients.) Among 41 abused borderline patients, 44% reported penetration, 54% reported ongoing sexual abuse, 66% reported abuse that was either ongoing or penetrating, 32% reported abuse that was both ongoing and penetrating, 32% reported sex with a parent, 54% reported sex with some nuclear family member, and 51% reported sexual abuse by at least two different people during their childhood. In fact, when we looked at our cohort with respect to those subjects who "only" experienced a single, nonpenetrating sexual event with someone other than a nuclear family member or relative, we found that two-thirds of our abused psychiatrically healthy control subjects and more than 50% of our abused depressed inpatients, but only 15% of our abused borderline inpatients, fell into this category.

Our goal was to categorize and study sexual abuse severity more precisely. In Study 3, we divided sexual abuse activity into three dimensions—perpetrator, frequency, and type—and we developed a severity scale based on these dimensions. We empirically chose seven items from the DIB and modeled them in a logistic regression to clarify the relationship between specific DIB items and parameters of sexual abuse severity, and also to determine which specific aspect of severity of sexual abuse might be the most significant predictor of some symptoms of BPD psychopathology.

Method

The selection of subjects follows the two studies described previously. In this study, we were interested only in subjects who reported a history of sexual abuse during childhood. The cohort consisted of 51 subjects: 41 borderline inpatients (by the DIB), 7 inpatients with major depressive disorder (by RDC), and 3 psychiatrically healthy control subjects.

To code severity of sexual abuse, we developed a sexual abuse severity scale (SXABSS) that ranked sexual abuse in three categories of severity. The categories were developed by an expert-panel method, whereby members of our research group were asked to sort severity of abuse into three categories, category 1 the least severe and 3 the most severe. Frequency of act, type of act, and specificity of perpetrator were considered when developing the three severity categories. Category 3 included subjects who reported ongoing penetrating sexual abuse either within or outside the nuclear family. Category 2 included subjects who had family sex as well as sex with persons other than nuclear family members. In this category the sexual abuse was either ongoing or penetrating, but not both, with the exception that a single nonpenetrating event involving a nuclear family member would also be classified here. Category 1 was confined to a single incident of nonpenetrating sexual activity that did not involve a nuclear family member (Silk et al. 1994).

Because of the sample size, we limited the number of DIB symptoms we studied. We accomplished this empirically by using a χ^2 test to examine univariate associations of the three categories of the SXABSS with each of the 29 items that are scored on the DIB. We created a subset of DIB items (DIB index) that included those DIB items that showed a "stairstep progressive" relationship across each of the three categories of the SXABSS in the univariate analyses: for a DIB item to be chosen, it needed to be endorsed by more subjects in category 3 (most severe) on the SXABSS than subjects in category 2 (intermediate severity), and by more subjects in category 2 than subjects in category 1 (least severe). This pattern of endorsement defined the stairstep progression. Seven DIB items were identified by this procedure. Positive responses on each of the seven items were summed, resulting in DIB index scores that ranged from 0 to 7.

Results

The sample was composed primarily of female borderline patients (36/51). Borderline subjects were significantly younger and reported most of the severe sexual abuse.

The DIB items of parasuicide, substance abuse, other impulse disturbance, chronic dysphoria, regression in therapy, conflict over giving and receiving care, and "causing staff splitting" all showed a stairstep progression difference across the three categories of severity of the SXABSS, and these seven DIB items made up our DIB index. Of interest is that of the three DIB symptoms found to be "general" predictors of sexual abuse in the Ogata et al. (1990b) study—derealization, promiscuity, and chronic dysphoria—only chronic dysphoria was empirically chosen in these univariate analyses.

Analysis of variance was used to test the differences between categories on the SXABSS and the DIB index score (range 0–7) as well as the between-category differences on the SXABSS and the total scaled DIB score (range 0–10). Analysis of variance among the three categories on the SXABSS and the DIB index score revealed a significant difference when all subjects ($N = 51$) were included in the analysis ($F = 8.70$, df = 2,48, $P < .001$) as well as when the analysis was restricted to the 36 female borderline patients ($F = 3.84$, df = 2,33, $P = .03$). Significant differences were found between each of the severity categories of the SXABSS among the larger sample of 51 subjects: category 1 versus category 2 ($P = .03$), category 1 versus category 3 ($P = .001$), and category 2 versus category 3 ($P = .03$). When the sample was limited to the female borderline patients, between-category differences on the SXABSS were significant when comparing the most severe with the least severe category—category 1 versus category 3 (P = .01). Analysis of variance to test differences between categories of severity on the SXABSS and the total DIB score was significant for the entire sample (F = 5.47, df = 2,48, P = .007), and significant differences were found between the least severe and the next two more severe categories: category 1 versus category 2 (P = .01) and category 1 versus category 3 (P = .003). This difference was not significant in the smaller female BPD sample. However, this result was expected, because the borderline subjects had, by definition, a DIB score of ≥ 7; and thus the possible range of DIB scores in this BPD sample was only 7–10, whereas the range in the larger sample was 0–10.

A second set of analyses was conducted to determine which of the three primary components of severity were significant predictors of 1) the specific DIB items that made up the index, 2) the DIB index total, and 3) the total scaled DIB score. Stepwise logistic regression was used to model each item, using the most severe predictors in each dimension of sexual abuse: abuse type (penetration), abuse duration (ongoing), and abuse perpetrator (parent). The variables were forced to be tested in the model until the residual variation was not significant at the .05 level. The regression was run twice, first with the full sample of 51 subjects and then with a smaller homogeneous sample of 36 female borderline patients (see Table 8–1). When all 51 subjects were included in the sample, ongoing sexual abuse predicted the DIB items of parasuicide, substance abuse, regression in therapy, the DIB index score, and the total scaled DIB score. Penetration predicted conflict over giving and receiving care. When the regressions were repeated with only the 36 female borderline patients, ongoing sexual abuse was the sole predictor, predicting parasuicide, regression in therapy, the DIB index score, and the total DIB scaled score. Age was significantly different between diagnostic groups, and age was added to the regression involving the entire sample. Age rather than ongoing sexual abuse then predicted substance abuse, but no other results were changed (Silk et al. 1994).

Repetition of sexual abuse—that is, abuse that is ongoing—appears to be the most frequent and powerful predictor of

Table 8–1. Results of logistic regressions to determine predictors of Diagnostic Interview for Borderlines (DIB) items selected by univariate analyses (χ^2, df = 1)

| DIB item | Predictors: penetration, ongoing, parent[a] | |
	Entire sample (*N* = 51)	Borderline females (*n* = 36)
Parasuicide	Ongoing (10.51)***	Ongoing (5.97)*
Substance abuse	Ongoing (6.12)**	—
Other impulses	—	—
Chronic dysphoria	—	—
Regression in therapy	Ongoing (6.12)**	Ongoing (4.12)*
Conflict over care	Penetration (5.03)*	—
Causes staff splitting	—	—
DIB index[b]	Ongoing (17.81)****	Ongoing (9.00)**
Scaled DIB score	Ongoing (13.05)****	Ongoing (4.58)*

[a]Penetration = sexual abuse that involved penetration; ongoing = ongoing sexual abuse; parent = sexual abuse by a parent.
[b]Sum of the 7 DIB items listed directly above.
*$P < .05$. **$P < .01$. ***$P < .001$. ****$P < .0001$.

a number of DIB items, particularly the tendency to parasuicide and the propensity to regress in therapeutic situations. Also of interest is that ongoing sexual abuse predicted the total DIB scaled score both in the full sample and in the sample of female borderline patients, where the range of scores is quite limited. Thus, if total DIB score is any measure of the degree or severity of "borderline-ness," then repetitive experiences of sexual abuse in childhood may be a predictor of the severity of the borderline illness.

The results of this study suggest that ongoing sexual abuse may predict symptoms that are well-known facets of interpersonal functioning among patients with BPD. Sexual abuse may particularly affect how the BPD patient appears in interpersonal and psychotherapeutic settings. Perhaps it is the duration of abuse and not abuse itself that fertilizes the soil in which future borderline patients' symptoms and behavior grow. Ongoing sexual abuse is a continuous, repetitive exposure to interpersonal trauma that damages one's attachments at an early age and profoundly affects one's capacity to attach in satisfying and safe ways in the future. These failures of attachment events appear to increase the risk of following a developmental pathway leading through distorted interpersonal development and on to adult character pathology. Severe or continuous abuse over years can also lead to a deep conviction that other people are unsafe and interested only in their own gratification, and hence to a malevolent object world.

STUDY 4: SEVERITY OF SEXUAL ABUSE AND FAMILY ENVIRONMENT

There is a common belief that the interplay between the experience of abuse and the family environment at the time of the abuse determines the psychological outcome in the victim. (It should be recalled that there were 3 psychiatrically healthy subjects who had a history of sexual abuse.) Further, the question has been raised repeatedly whether abuse causes pathological family relationships or whether abuse results from those pathological relationships. Fromuth (1986) believed that it was more the lack of parental supportiveness and not the sexual abuse itself that determined the later poor adjustment in certain victims of childhood sexual abuse.

Nash et al. (1993) administered a family functioning self-report instrument to abused and nonabused subjects to assess the relationship between family dysfunction and symptoms assessed from the MMPI and the Rorschach. Although both family dysfunction and sexual abuse were associated with psychopathology, covariation for recalled family pathology eliminated most of the differences between the abused and nonabused samples (although several remained—hypochondriasis and paranoia subscale differences on the MMPI and a self-perception cluster on the Rorschach).

Although the question of relative influence on future psychopathology of family dysfunction and sexual abuse is difficult to determine, it is useful to explore how borderline patients and how abused patients (both borderline and nonborderline) retrospectively view the environment of their families of origin. There are many more people who are sexually abused than who become borderline, and at least 25% of borderline patients do not report abuse (Paris and Zweig-Frank 1992); thus the question is raised whether the BPD diagnosis and sexual abuse would predict similar family-of-origin environments. Perry and Herman (1993) suggest that there are a number of aspects of childhood family environment that could contribute to the development of a borderline disorder: verbal abuse, parental psychopathology, lack of a protective environment or atmosphere that supports people's confiding in each other, grossly inappropriate parental behavior (e.g., sexual abuse), and a generally chaotic home environment. It makes logical sense that the more nurturing and supportive a family environment is, the more the environment should be able to buffer the effects of childhood trauma.

Studies that have explored the family-of-origin environment of borderline patients have found the parents in these families to be either neglectful or overinvolved (Gunderson 1984; Gunderson and Englund 1981). Gunderson et al. (1980) found that the most distinctive pattern in the families of borderline patients was parental neglect of the children. Intrafamilial sexual abuse, it seems, is an example of simultaneous neglect and overinvolvement.

Few empirical studies have explored how borderline patients view their parents or their parental environment. Paris and Frank (Frank and Paris 1981; Paris and Zweig-Frank 1993), using the Parental Bonding Index (Parker 1983) in a series of studies, found that in some studies, fathers were perceived as less caring and approving, and in others, mothers were perceived that way. Although there is some discrepancy across studies, most studies of borderline patients' perceptions of their parents propose a pattern of biparental failure and neglect (Goldberg et al. 1985; Links et al. 1990; Paris and Zweig-Frank 1993; Zanarini et al. 1989). In a previous study, some of the authors of this chapter (Baker et al. 1992) used the Adjective Checklist (ACL) (Gough and Heilbrun 1983) to assess borderline patients' retrospective perceptions of their parents. We studied seven ACL scales: Favorable, Unfavorable, Nurturance, Critical Parent, Nurturing Parent (which we called Conscientiousness), Aggression, and Dominance. Although we undertook the study to explore whether borderline patients had a tendency to split representations of their parents into one good parent and one bad parent, we found that rather than split these representations, borderline patients had a significantly greater tendency to depict both their parents in more negative terms than did either depressed inpatients or psychiatrically healthy control subjects. A significant portion of the variance in the father scores related to sexual abuse.

In another earlier study (Ogata et al. 1990a), an author of this chapter and others explored retrospective recollections of the childhood family environment of adult borderline patients by comparing 24 borderline patients with 18 depressed nonborderline patients on the Family Environment Scale (FES) (Moos and Moos 1981). The FES is made up of 90 true-false items and has good internal consistency and test-retest reliability. The FES has 10 subscales divided into three dimensions. The Relationships dimension consists of the subscales Conflict, Expressiveness, and Cohesion. The System Maintenance dimension consists of the subscales Organization and Control. The Personal Growth dimension consists of Independence, Achievement Orientation, Intellectual-Cultural Orientation, Active-Recreation Orientation, and Moral-Religious Orientation. In this study, FES scores were considered for the family of origin during two periods: when subjects were ages 0–12, and when subjects were ages 13–18. For the 0- to 12-year-old time span, the borderline patients scored their families lower on Cohesion than did the depressed subjects. For the 13- to 18-year-old time span, the borderline patients scored their families lower on Cohesion and higher on Conflict than did the depressed patients. Data with respect to a history of sexual abuse were not considered at that time.

The FES has been used in a number of studies to explore the family environment of sexually abused persons. Wilson (1982) compared the family environments of 30 families in treatment because sexual abuse had been reported in the family with 30 families of the faculty of Northwestern College of St. Paul, Minnesota. She found that the FES subscales significantly associated with the sexual abuse families were lower Intellectual-Cultural Orientation, higher Conflict, lower Moral-Religious Emphasis, and lower Cohesion. Long and Jackson (1991) used five FES scales to compare 146 sexually abused persons who had been exposed to single perpetrators in their lifetime with 15 sexually abused persons who had been exposed to multiple perpetrators in their lifetime. The research group found that the families of those abused by multiple perpetrators were significantly lower in Cohesion, Expressiveness, and Control and significantly higher in Conflict. Ray et al. (1991) found no FES scale differences in subjects who had been exposed to intrafamilial versus extrafamilial sexual abuse, but they found that all those abused had families with significantly lower scores on Cohesion, Independence, Organization, Active-Recreational Orientation, and Moral-Religious Emphasis. None of these studies, however, looked at both sexual abuse and diagnosis, and thus none of these studies could address the issue of whether diagnosis and sexual abuse affected different FES subscale scores.

Method

Subjects were identified as above, and all were given the FES.

Results

There were 67 subjects in the study (37 with BPD by the DIB, 16 with MDD by RDC, and 14 well-screened psychiatrically healthy control subjects). Thirty-seven subjects reported sexual abuse on the FEI (28 with BPD, 6 with MDD, and 3 control subjects). Borderline subjects were significantly younger than the other two groups ($F = 11.3$, df = 2,64, $P < .0001$) and had experienced significantly more sexual abuse than the other two groups ($\chi^2 = 14.8$, df = 2, $P < .001$).

A series of multiple linear regressions was run; each of the 10 FES subscales was used as the dependent variable, and diagnosis, gender, and a number of measures of sexual abuse severity were used as the independent or predictor variables. The sexual abuse measures used were any history of sexual abuse, penetrating sexual abuse, ongoing sexual abuse, sexual abuse that was either penetrating or ongoing, and sexual abuse that was both penetrating and ongoing. Of interest is that the scales and the periods that were significantly different in the borderline patients (compared with the depressed inpatients) in the Ogata et al. (1990a) study remained the same subscales and periods predicted by diagnosis rather than by a sexual abuse parameter (see Table 8–2). In the current study, the diagnosis of BPD predicted lower Cohesion in both periods, lower Expressiveness during childhood, less Active-Recreational Orientation during both childhood and adolescence, less Independence and less Intellectual-Cultural Orientation during adolescence, and higher Conflict in teenage years. In addition to the diagnosis, female gender also predicted higher Conflict during the teenage period. Any type of sexual abuse predicted less Expressiveness during adolescence.

Table 8–2. Multiple regression of Family Environment Scale (FES) subscales with diagnosis, gender, and severity of sexual abuse measures as predictors

Type of subscale by prediction	Age group (years)	
	0–12	**13–18**
Subscales predicted lower by borderline diagnosis	Cohesion (20.7)[a]**** Active-Recreational Orientation (6.71)** Expressiveness (9.29)***	Cohesion (29.5)**** Active-Recreational Orientation (4.33)* Independence (4.52)* Intellectual-Cultural Orientation (8.42)***
Subscales predicted higher by borderline diagnosis	—	Conflict (6.41)[b]***
Subscales predicted lower by sexual abuse measures	Independence (5.95)[c]* Moral-Religious Orientation (5.32)[c]* Organization (10.8)[d]*** Intellectual-Cultural Orientation (4.75)[e]*	Expressiveness (7.25)[f]** Moral-Religious Orientation (4.72)[c]* Organization (10.44)[d]***

[a]F values are in parentheses.
[b]Female gender also predicted conflict here.
[c]Penetrating and ongoing sexual abuse.
[d]Penetrating or ongoing sexual abuse.
[e]Ongoing sexual abuse.
[f]Any sexual abuse.
*$P < .05$. **$P < .01$. ***$P < .005$. ****$P < .001$.

Sexual abuse that was penetrating and ongoing predicted less Independence during childhood and less Moral-Religious Orientation during both childhood and adolescence. Sexual abuse that was either penetrating or ongoing predicted lower familial Organization during both childhood and adolescence. Ongoing sexual abuse predicted less Intellectual-Cultural Orientation during childhood.

The multiple regressions, then, even when accounting for sexual abuse, did not change the scales that the borderline diagnosis predicted in the study by Ogata et al. (1990a) when sexual abuse was not considered in the analysis. Cohesion, Conflict, and Expressiveness, three of the five scales predicted by diagnosis, fall into the Relationships dimension of the FES. Of further interest is that of the five subscales predicted by the occurrence of sexual abuse during childhood or adolescence, three of the five belong to the Personal Growth dimension of the FES.

This study suggests that diagnosis and sexual abuse may predict different family environments, implying that there may be at least two pathways to BPD. The Personal Growth dimension may relate particularly to people's self-esteem, goals, and identity, and that dimension appears to be affected by both diagnosis and history of sexual abuse. Diagnosis also seems to affect the dimension of relationships, and again—thinking about BPD as essentially a disorder of interpersonal relationships—this study suggests that low self-esteem and a lack of feeling connected to one's family (cohesion) and a failure to have a milieu in which to express one's concerns (expressiveness) can lead to a feeling of alienation and ultimately to conflict with others.

CLINICAL RELEVANCE

These four studies may lead us to a clearer clinical picture of the borderline patient, particularly the one who has been sexually abused. When Herman and van der Kolk (1987) first proposed the idea of sexual abuse as a significant etiological factor in BPD, there was some hope that perhaps viewing borderline patients as victims of abuse, rather than as manipulative patients destined to make therapists' lives difficult, might reduce some of the negative countertransference directed at these patients. In some ways this has been true, but advocates of false memory syndrome, as well as the therapists who think that all borderline patients must have been abused, have introduced new controversies and confounding variables into the treatment.

CHILDHOOD FAMILIAL ENVIRONMENT AND EXPERIENCES

Nonetheless, our research begins to help us draw a rough, broad portrait of the developmental experiences of borderline patients. Borderline patients appear to come from families where their emotional needs are not met and their movement toward independence and personal growth is not supported. The family lacks cohesion, and children are not supported in their need to express their feelings. Expressing feelings does not lead to an empathic and supportive response, but perhaps to criticism or blame or just to no response at all. Proper attachment to primary caregivers is clearly not established. Safety with respect to the expression of one's feelings does not exist, and it is in this familial context that the person experiences either intra- or extrafamilial sexual abuse.

In either instance, however, the abuse victim is unable to turn to the family for support, and lacking this avenue to work through the emotional pain, the victim dissociates, splits off the pain, and removes herself psychologically from the emotional and perhaps physical pain. In adolescence, the future BPD patient struggles, mostly through conflict with the family, to gain some independence, despite the fact that she has few tools with which to attain independence and little confidence or self-esteem with which to help move herself in that direction. Pseudo-adult behavior ensues, with sexual activity and substance abuse that recreate the sexual and dissociative situations of earlier periods of her childhood. Hurt again, and taken advantage of in the pseudo-adult impulsive situations, the victim of repeated abuse has reinforced the idea of the world as a cold, malevolent place. Borderline patients feel that the people to whom they get close often abandon them (or at least do not support them) emotionally, and they both wish for close contact and fear experiencing the pain and the fear of abandonment that accompanies any attachment.

PSYCHOTHERAPY WITH THE ABUSED BORDERLINE PATIENT

Sexual abuse presents a dilemma for the psychotherapist who treats the abused patient. The patient sometimes experiences the therapist not as a protector, but as a threat. This transferential expectation may then contribute to negative therapeutic reactions in the therapy of the borderline patient (Herman 1992), for the more the patient becomes attached to the therapist, the more dangerous the therapist becomes to him or her. This view of the therapist as a potential abuser may account for periods of regression or increased acting-out behavior following times when, in the therapist's opinion, there has been progress in the therapy. Thinking in terms of reenactments of sexual abuse in the treatment helps explain some behavior previously understood only generically as difficulty with closeness and distance. These reenactments involve expectations of malevolence and harm from the therapist as the patient grows closer to the therapist, as well as an underlying feeling that the therapist is really not interested in the personal growth of the patient. Attachment is both longed for and feared, and these complex conflicts often manifest themselves in repeated indirect requests for help (Zanarini and Frankenburg 1994).

OTHER CONSIDERATIONS

Our portrait has obviously ignored other factors, including biological dimensions that may be pertinent (Siever and Davis 1991; Silk 1994). Differential responses of persons with varying genotypes to particular family environments have been demonstrated in behavioral genetic research (Bergeman et al. 1988). However, the best behavioral genetic data on personality development suggest that in addition to genotype, both shared and unshared environmental experiences contribute to the emergence of negative affect, impulsivity, interpersonal hostility, and other features of personality potentially relevant to BPD (Bergeman et al. 1993; Tellegen et al. 1988). It is quite plausible that the development of BPD requires the accumulation of multiple risks, perhaps including varying combinations of temperament, adverse family environment, and sexual abuse or other trauma (Nigg and Goldsmith 1994). Our data are consistent with the idea that there are at least two developmental pathways to BPD. Ongoing severe sexual abuse may be such a strong risk factor for BPD that a wide range of biological predispositions give rise to BPD in the presence of such trauma, whereas BPD patients who have not been traumatized may have a higher loading of risks in the domains of biological predisposition and general adverse family environment. Although this portrait is somewhat speculative, the research on retrospective recall of sexual abuse in BPD provides a powerful explanatory hypothesis for the features of psychopathology that previously might have seemed contradictory or inexplicable. Such data can help the field move beyond personal reactions to a careful scientific model of the role of abuse in the development of this troubling disorder.

REFERENCES

American Psychiatric Association: Diagnostic and Statistical Manual of Mental Disorders, 3rd Edition, Revised. Washington, DC, American Psychiatric Press, 1987

Baker L, Silk KR, Westen D, et al: Malevolence, splitting, and parental ratings by borderlines. J Nerv Ment Dis 180:258–264, 1992

Barends A, Westen D, Byers S, et al: Assessing affect-tone of relationship paradigms from TAT and interview data. Psychological Assessment 2:239–332, 1990

Benjamin J, Silk KR, Lohr N, et al: The relationship between borderline personality disorder and the anxiety disorders. Am J Orthopsychiatry 59:461–467, 1989

Bergeman CS, Plomin R, McClearn GE, et al: Genotype-environment interaction in personality development: identical twins reared apart. Psychol Aging 3:399–406, 1988

Bergeman CS, Chipuer HM, Plomin R, et al: Genetic and environmental effects on openness to experience, agreeableness, and conscientiousness: an adoption/twin study. J Pers 61:159–179, 1993

Brewin CR, Andrews B, Gotlib IH: Psychopathology and early experience: a reappraisal of retrospective reports. Psychol Bull 113:82–98, 1993

Briere J, Conte J: Self-reported amnesia for abuse in adults. Journal of Traumatic Stress 6:21–31, 1993

Briere J, Runtz M: Suicidal thoughts and behaviours in former sexual abuse victims. Canadian Journal of Behavioural Sciences 18:413–423, 1986

Briere J, Conte J: Self-reported amnesia for abuse in adults. Journal of Traumatic Stress 6:21–31, 1993

Browne A, Finkelhor D: Impact of child sexual abuse: a review of the literature. Psychol Bull 99:66–77, 1986

Bruhn AR, Last J: Earliest childhood memories: four theoretical perspectives. J Pers Assess 46:119–127, 1982

Carmen E, Reiker PP, Mills T: Victims of violence and psychiatric illness. Am J Psychiatry 141:378–383, 1984

Cornell DG, Silk KR, Ludolph PS, et al: Test-retest reliability of the Diagnostic Interview for Borderlines. Arch Gen Psychiatry 40:1307–1310, 1983

Davis P: Repression and the inaccessibility of affective memories. J Pers Soc Psychol 53:585– 593, 1987

Dittburner TL, Persinger MA: Intensity of amnesia during hypnosis is positively correlated with estimated prevalence of sexual abuse and alien abductions: implication for the false memory syndrome. Percept Mot Skills 77:895–898, 1993

Exner JE: The Rorschach: A Comprehensive System. New York, Wiley, 1993

Frank H, Paris J: Recollections of family experience in borderline patients. Arch Gen Psychiatry 38:1031–1034, 1981

Frankel FH: Adult reconstruction of childhood events in the multiple personality literature. Am J Psychiatry 150:954–958, 1993

Fromuth ME: The relationship of childhood sexual abuse with later psychological and sexual adjustment in a sample of college women. Child Abuse Negl 10:5–15, 1986

Gardner RA: Sex Abuse Hysteria: Salem Witch Trials Revisited. Cresskill, NJ, Creative Therapeutics, 1991

Gold LJ, Silk KR: Exploring the borderline personality disorder-major affective disorder interface, in Borderline Personality Disorder: Etiology and Treatment. Edited by Paris J. Washington, DC, American Psychiatric Press, 1993, pp 39–66

Goldberg RL, Mann LS, Wise TN, et al: Parental qualities as perceived by borderline personality disorders. Hillside Journal of Clinical Psychiatry 7:134–140, 1985

Gough HG, Heilbrun AB: The Adjective Check List Manual. Palo Alto, CA: Consulting Psychologists Press, 1983

Green AH: Dimensions of psychological trauma in abused children. J Am Acad Child Adolesc Psychiatry 22:231–237, 1983

Grinfeld MJ, Reisman J: Childhood sex abuse memories haunt victims, divide experts. Psychiatric Times 10:1, 5–6, August 1993

Gross J: Suit asks, does "memory therapy" heal or harm? The New York Times, April 8, 1994, pp 1, B16

Gunderson JG: Borderline Personality Disorder. Washington, DC, American Psychiatric Press, 1984

Gunderson JG, Englund DW: Characterizing the families of borderlines. Psychiatr Clin North Am 4:159–168, 1981

Gunderson JG, Phillips KA: A current view of the interface between borderline personality disorder and depression. Am J Psychiatry 148:967–975, 1991

Gunderson JG, Sabo AN: The phenomenological and conceptual interface between borderline personality disorder and PTSD. Am J Psychiatry 150:19–27, 1993

Gunderson JG, Kerr J, Englund D: The families of borderlines: a comparative study. Arch Gen Psychiatry 37:27–33, 1980

Gunderson JG, Kolb JE, Austin V: The Diagnostic Interview for Borderline patients. Am J Psychiatry 138:896–903, 1981

Hathaway SR, McKinley JC: Minnesota Multiphasic Personality Inventory—2. Minneapolis, MN, University of Minnesota, 1989

Herman JL: Trauma and Recovery. New York, Basic Books, 1992

Herman JL, Schatzow E: Recovery and verification of memories of childhood sexual trauma. Psychoanalytic Psychology 4:1–14, 1987

Herman JL, van der Kolk BA: Traumatic antecedents of borderline personality disorder, in Psychological Trauma. Edited by van der Kolk BA. Washington, DC, American Psychiatric Press, 1987, pp 111–126

Herman JL, Russell D, Trocki K: Long-term effects of incestuous abuse in childhood. Am J Psychiatry 143:1293–1296, 1986

Herman JL, Perry JC, van der Kolk BA: Childhood trauma in borderline personality disorder. Am J Psychiatry 146:490–495, 1989

Jacobson A, Richardson B: Assault experiences of 100 psychiatric inpatients: evidence of the need for routine inquiry. Am J Psychiatry 144: 908–913, 1987

Jacobson E: The Self and the Object World. New York, International Universities Press, 1964

Jason J, Williams SL, Burton A, et al: Epidemiologic differences between sexual and physical child abuse. JAMA 247:3344–3348, 1982

Jones DP, McGraw JM: Reliable and fictitious accounts of sexual abuse of children. Journal of Interpersonal Violence 2:27–45, 1987

Kendall-Tackett K, Williams LM, Finkelhor D: Impact of sexual abuse on children: a review and synthesis of recent empirical findings. Psychol Bull 113:164–180, 1993

Kernberg O: Borderline Conditions and Pathological Narcissism. New York, Jason Aronson, 1975

Kernberg O: Object-Relations Theory and Clinical Psychoanalysis. New York, Jason Aronson, 1976

Kluft RP: Introduction, in Incest Related Syndromes of Adult Psychopathology. Edited by Kluft RP. Washington, DC, American Psychiatric Press, 1990, pp 1–10

Lewinsohn PM, Rosenbaum M: Recall of parental behavior by acute depressives, remitted depressives, and nondepressives. J Pers Soc Psychol 52:611–619, 1987

Links PS, Boiago I, Huxley G, et al: Sexual abuse and biparental failure as etiologic models in borderline personality disorder, in Family Environment and Borderline Personality Disorder. Edited by Links PS. American Psychiatric Press, Washington, DC, 1990, pp 107–120

Loftus EF: The reality of repressed memories. Am Psychol 48:518–537, 1993

Long PJ, Jackson JL: Children sexually abused by multiple perpetrators. Journal of Interpersonal Violence 6:147–159, 1991

Lynn SJ, Rhue JW: Fantasy proneness: hypnosis, developmental antecedents, and psychopathology. Am Psychol 43:35–44, 1988

Masterson JF: Psychotherapy of the Borderline Adult. New York, Brunner/Mazel, 1976

Mayman M: Early memories and character structure. Journal of Projective Technique and Personality Assessment 32:303–316, 1968

Mayman M, Faris M: Early memories as expressions of relationship paradigms. Am J Orthopsychiatry 30:507–520, 1960

Moos R, Moos B: Family Environment Scale Manual. Palo Alto, CA: Consulting Psychologists Press, 1981

Nash MR, Hulsey TL, Sexton MC, et al: Long-term sequelae of childhood sexual abuse: perceived family environment, psychopathology, and dissociation. J Consult Clin Psychol 61: 276–283, 1993

Nigg JT, Goldsmith HH: Genetics of personality disorders: perspectives from personality and psychopathology research. Psychol Bull 115:346–380, 1994

Nigg JT, Silk KR, Westen D, et al: Object representations in the early memories of sexually abused borderline patients. Am J Psychiatry 148:864–869, 1991

Nigg JT, Lohr NE, Westen D, et al: Malevolent object representations in borderline personality disorder and major depression. J Abnorm Psychol 101:61–67, 1992

Ofshe R: Inadvertent hypnosis during interrogation: false confessions due to dissociative state: mis-identified multiple personality and the satanic cult hypothesis. Int J Clin Exp Hypn 40:125–156, 1992

Ofshe R, Waters E: Making monsters. Society 4–16, March-April 1993

Olafson E, Corwin D, Summit R: Modern history of child sexual abuse and awareness: cycles of discovery and suppression. Child Abuse Negl 17:7–24, 1993

Ogata SN: A comparison of early family histories of borderline and depressed patients (abstract). Dissertation Abstracts International 49(9-B):4040, 1989

Ogata SN, Silk KR, Goodrich S: The childhood experience of the borderline patient, in Family Environment and Borderline Personality Disorder. Edited by Links PS. Washington, DC, American Psychiatric Press, 1990a, pp 85–103

Ogata SN, Silk KR, Goodrich S, et al: Childhood sexual and physical abuse in adult patients with borderline personality disorder. Am J Psychiatry 147:1008–1013, 1990b

Paris J, Zweig-Frank H: A critical review of childhood sexual abuse in the etiology of borderline personality disorder. Can J Psychiatry 37:125–128, 1992

Paris J, Zweig-Frank H: Parental bonding in borderline personality disorder, in Borderline Personality Disorder: Etiology and Treatment. Edited by Paris J. Washington, DC, American Psychiatric Press, 1993, pp 141–159

Parker G: Parental Overprotection: A Risk Factor in Psycho-Social Development. New York, Grune and Stratton, 1983

Perry JC, Herman JL: Trauma and defense in the etiology of borderline personality disorder, in Borderline Personality Disorder: Etiology and Treatment. Edited by Paris J. Washington, DC, American Psychiatric Press, 1993, pp 123–139

Ray KC, Jackson JL, Townsley RM: Family environments of victims of intrafamilial and extrafamilial chld sexual abuse. Journal of Family Violence 6:365–374, 1991

Rosenberg M: Society and the Adolescent Self-Image. Princeton, NJ, Princeton University Press, 1965

Russell DEH: Sexual Exploitation: Rape, Child Sexual Abuse and Workplace Harassment. Beverly Hills, CA, Sage, 1984

Sandler J, Rosenblatt B: The concept of the representational study of the world. Psychoanal Study Child 17:128–145, 1961

Sedney MA, Brooks B: Factors associated with a history of childhood sexual experiences in a nonclinical female population. J Am Acad Child Adolesc Psychiatry 23:215–218, 1984

Siever LJ, Davis KL: A psychobiological perspective on the personality disorders. Am J Psychiatry 148:1647–1658, 1991

Silk KR: Implications of biological research for clinical practice with borderline patients, in Biological and Neurobehavioral Studies of Borderline Personality Disorder. Edited by Silk KR. Washington, DC, American Psychiatric Press, 1994, pp 227–240

Silk KR, Karle B, Lohr NE, et al: Sexual abuse and family environment in borderline personality disorder. Paper presented at the 146th annual meeting of the American Psychiatric Association, San Francisco, CA, May 22–27, 1993

Silk KR, Lee S, Hill EM, et al: Borderline symptoms and severity of sexual abuse. Paper presented at the 147th annual meeting of the American Psychiatric Association, Philadelphia, PA, May 21–26, 1994

Spitzer RL, Endicott JE, Robins E: Research Diagnostic Criteria (RDC) for a Selected Group of Functional Disorders, 2nd Edition. New York, Biometrics Research, New York State Psychiatric Institute, 1975

Stone MH: Borderline syndromes: a consideration of subtypes and an overview: directions for research. Psychiatr Clin North Am 4:3–13, 1981

Taylor JA: Early recollections as a projective technique: a review of some recent validation studies. Journal of Individual Psychology 30:213–218, 1975

Tellegen A, Lykken DT, Bouchard TJ, et al: Personality similarity in twins reared apart and together. J Pers Soc Psychol 54:1031–1039, 1988

Westen D: Toward a revised theory of borderline object relations: implications of empirical research. Int J Psychoanal 71:661–693, 1990

Westen D, Lohr NE, Silk KR, et al: Object relations and social cognition in borderlines, major depressives and normals: a TAT analysis. Psychological Assessment 2:355–364, 1990a

Westen D, Ludolph P, Misle B, et al: Physical and sexual abuse in adolescent girls with borderline personality disorder. Am J Orthopsychiatry 60:55–66, 1990b

Williams LM: Adult memories of childhood abuse: preliminary findings from a longitudinal study. The Advisor 5:19–20, 1992

Wilson K: Child sexual abuse: a comparison of the attitudes and environments of abusing and non-abusing families (abstract). Dissertation Abstracts International 43(2-B):539, 1982

Zanarini MC, Frankenburg FR: Emotional hypochondriasis, hyperbole, and the borderline patient. J Psychotherapy Practice Research 3:25–36, 1994

Zanarini MC, Gunderson JG, Marino MF, et al: Childhood experiences of borderline patients. Compr Psychiatry 30:18–25, 1989

Chapter 9

Neurological Vulnerability and Trauma in Borderline Personality Disorder

Catherine Rising Kimble, M.D., Godehard Oepen, M.D.,
Elizabeth Weinberg, M.D., Amy A. Williams, B.S.,
and Mary C. Zanarini, Ed.D.

Many symptoms of patients with borderline personality disorder (BPD)—such as impulsivity, irritability, low frustration tolerance, perceptual and memory distortions, and affective instability—sufficiently resemble the symptomatology of brain-injured patients to suggest that these traits might be neurologically mediated. Rather than contradicting evidence for the role of early childhood abuse in BPD (Herman et al. 1989; Links et al. 1988; Ogata et al. 1990; Shearer et al. 1990; Westen et al. 1990; Zanarini et al. 1989b), studying subtle developmental or acquired neurological dysfunction and its relationship to BPD may help elucidate the etiology of the disorder and the clinical understanding of borderline patients.

The interplay of biological injury and behavior was described in Rutter's research (1982) on "minimal brain dysfunction" (MBD) and its possible role in the development of later psychopathology. An organic hypothesis of BPD itself was originally proposed by Andrulonis and colleagues (Andrulonis and Vogel 1984; Andrulonis et al. 1981, 1982). In a chart review study, 14% of nonschizotypal borderline patients had a history of head

Supported in part by National Institute of Mental Health grant MH47588 to Dr. Zanarini.

165

trauma, encephalitis, or epilepsy, and 26% had a history of attention deficit disorder (ADD) and/or a learning disability. Borderline patients were significantly more likely than control subjects with affective disorders (but not schizophrenia) to have a history of organic disturbance (both subcategories combined) as well as a history of head trauma, encephalitis, or epilepsy. In addition, these authors found that a significantly higher percentage of male than of female borderline subjects had a history of organic disturbance (52% vs. 29%) as well as a history of ADD or learning disability (40% vs. 14%).

Soloff and Millward (1983) proposed a neurobehavioral model, postulating that BPD might result as a developmental adaptation to childhood brain dysfunction that impairs the child's integrative and inhibitory capacities. They concluded, however, that their data did not support such a model. Their data failed to demonstrate significant differences in comparing 45 borderline patients (83% women) with 32 patients meeting criteria for major depression and 42 patients meeting criteria for schizophrenia. Their study compared routine developmental histories, including problems of childbirth, childhood illnesses, developmental milestones, learning difficulties, and "hyperactivity." Excluded were patients with known substance abuse or dependence, central nervous system (CNS) deficits, organic brain syndromes, mental retardation, and seizure disorders. Although in the total sample they found prominent learning disabilities (16 patients having difficulty with reading, 8 with writing, and 12 with mathematics), these were not discriminating for borderline patients. In addition, they found no significant difference for hyperactivity or any other neurological abnormality studied. At the same time, a trend for prematurity or low birth rate was observed in their borderline group. In contrast, they did find higher rates of parental separation and loss, as well as overinvolved mothers and underinvolved fathers.

Fyer et al. (1988) did a retrospective study on 180 inpatients with BPD by DSM-III criteria (American Psychiatric Association 1980) that also supported the concept of the relevance of "organicity" in borderline patients. Borderline patients had a significantly lower rate of psychotic disorders and a significantly higher rate of unspecified "organic diagnoses." Recently, Van

Reekum et al. (1993) found results consistent with the concept of a subgroup of impaired organic borderline patients. In a case-controlled retrospective chart review of 48 primarily male veterans with BPD and 50 age-matched control subjects with mixed psychiatric disorders, a substantially higher rate of brain injuries was found among the patients with BPD (81%) than among the control subjects (22%).

In our previous retrospective study (Zanarini et al. 1994), we examined available neurological data in a retrospective chart review of 162 criteria-defined borderline patients and 134 control subjects with other personality disorders. Three findings emerged from this study. First, some form of subtle neurological dysfunction was quite common among our sample of borderline patients. Second, this dysfunction was not specific to borderline patients; it was also common in control subjects with near-neighbor Axis II disorders. Third, no specific relationship could be found between variables of reported abuse or other childhood experiences examined and neurological impairment in adult borderline patients.

Despite some (mostly retrospective) studies, the evidence for, and potential significance of, neurological dysfunction in borderline patients appears quite controversial and nonspecific. It is possible that subtle neurological impairment may predispose to behavioral abnormalities in borderline patients or in patients with personality disorders in general. Or subtle neurological injury may be the result of abuse or of self-destructive acts such as substance abuse. The purposes of our study were 1) to examine prospectively the frequency of variables suggesting brain dysfunction in borderline patients compared with control subjects who had personality disorders and 2) to assess the relationship between these frequencies and reported rates of pathological childhood experiences in the same group of patients. Our goal was to begin to understand the relative importance and possible interaction of both neurology and pathological childhood experiences in the development of borderline personality. To our knowledge, ours is the first prospective study that involves direct patient interviews to examine both neurological factors and trauma in the same group of borderline patients. The following study represents preliminary results of an ongoing prospective long-term follow-up study.

We focused on the following three questions: First, do border-line patients have more evidence of neurodevelopmental or acquired neurological impairment than patients with other Axis II disorders, and if so, which forms of neurological impairment are more prominent? Second, do neurologically vulnerable border-line patients differ with respect to reported rates of childhood abuse and neglect? Third, can a model that considers both pathological childhood experiences and neurological dysfunction adequately discriminate patients meeting criteria for BPD from those meeting criteria for other Axis II disorders?

METHODS

The current study involves pilot data taken from an ongoing prospective study of the longitudinal course of BPD—the McLean Study of Adult Development (MSAD). The diagnostic and childhood-history methodology of this study, which involves 300 inpatients at McLean Hospital, is basically the same as that used in earlier studies by our research group. (For further details, see Zanarini et al., Chapter 3, and Dubo et al., Chapter 7, this volume.) In the current study, age range was quite restricted: 18–35 years at the time of index admission.

Neurodevelopmental histories were obtained by a third team of interviewers. All were physicians blind to diagnostic and childhood history data. The MSAD Neurodevelopmental History and Temporolimbic Interview (MSAD NHTI) is composed of a semistructured interview and a neurological examination that assess 1) variables suggesting neurodevelopmental delay and 2) variables suggesting acquired CNS insults.

Eight variables were examined that might suggest neurodevelopmental delay: reported alcohol or drug exposure during the mother's pregnancy, evidence for high-risk or complicated pregnancy or birth (miscarriages before the patient's birth, vaginal bleeding during the mother's pregnancy, prematurity, prolonged labor, and low birth weight), history of developmental speech and language disorders, history of developmental reading or writing disorders, history of developmental arithmetic disorders, history of gross motor coordination impairment, history of fine motor coordination impairment, and symptoms of childhood attention deficit/hyperactivity disorder (ADHD). Four variables suggesting acquired injury were also assessed: history of physical stress in infancy, one or more CNS insults (known head injury or blackouts from drug and alcohol use), history of childhood seizures, and history of adult seizures. We also used this interview to screen for (but we do not report on) symptoms of temporal lobe epilepsy, endocrine disorders, and chronobiological abnormalities, and we also assessed (but do not report on) "soft signs," using a standardized neurological examination based on previously published methods (Woods et al. 1986).

Between-group comparisons involving categorical data were tested for significance with the χ^2 statistic corrected for continuity (Yates' correction). Between-group comparisons involving continuous data were computed with independent t tests. Neurological variables shown to be possibly related to BPD—either in past publications or in our own recent evaluation—were combined into a composite variable termed *vulnerable CNS substrate*: alcohol or drug exposure during mother's pregnancy, speech and language disturbance, head injury, seizure history, and symptoms of ADHD. A forced-entry logistic regression was also conducted to determine the relative predictive power for the borderline diagnosis of the 12 pathological childhood experiences studied, as well as the composite variable pertaining to CNS vulnerability.

RESULTS

In total, 63 female inpatients were interviewed; 40 patients met our research criteria for BPD, and 2 patients met DSM-III-R (American Psychiatric Association 1987) criteria for another Axis II disorder. Table 9–1 compares the prevalence of the neurological variables studied in borderline patients and in control subjects with personality disorders. No individual neurological variable discriminated significantly between patients with BPD and patients with other Axis II disorders. However, there were trends toward more common occurrence of childhood speech and language disturbance and of CNS insults in borderline subjects than in control subjects. In addition, our composite variable measuring "vulnerable CNS substrate" was significantly more common among borderline patients than among control subjects.

There were high rates of abuse and neglect in both BPD and control groups. Comparison with χ^2 analyses revealed no significant differences between borderline and control groups for any of these four abuse or eight neglect variables.

In Table 9–2, the prevalence of pathological childhood experiences in borderline patients with and without a vulnerable CNS substrate are reported. Only verbal abuse was significantly more prevalent in the vulnerable CNS substrate subgroup than in the borderline group without vulnerable CNS substrate. Although not significant, it is notable that sexual abuse was the only variable seen substantially more frequently in the subgroup without the vulnerable CNS substrate than in the subgroup with this trait (100.0% versus 74.3%).

A logistic regression was then performed, using the composite variable representing vulnerable CNS substrate and all individ-

Table 9–1. Prevalence of neurological variables in borderline patients and control subjects with personality disorders

Variable	% BPD	% OPD
Maternal alcohol/drug use	45.0	30.4
Complications of birth/pregnancy	32.5	21.7
Physical stress in infancy	17.5	26.1
Developmental speech/language impairment*	32.5	8.7
Developmental reading/writing impairment	22.5	21.7
Developmental arithmetic impairment	40.0	26.1
Developmental gross motor impairment	17.5	13.0
Developmental fine motor impairment	12.5	0.0
Diagnosis of childhood ADHD	12.5	4.3
One or more CNS insults*	67.5	39.1
Childhood seizure disorder	7.5	13.0
Adult seizure disorder	22.5	8.7
Composite vulnerable CNS substrate**	87.5	47.8

Note. BPD = borderline personality disorder. OPD = other personality disorder. ADHD = attention deficit/hyperactivity disorder. CNS = central nervous system.
*Trend at $P < .10$. **Statistically significant at $P < .01$.

ual childhood variables as independent variables. This model predicted a diagnosis correctly in 76.2% of the cases (χ^2 = 28.1, df = 13, P = .0089); 87.5% of the borderline patients, but only 64.7% of the Axis II control subjects, were correctly classified. In this analysis, only two variables were found to be significant. More specifically, patients with suggested neurological vulnerability were 6.4 times more likely to have met criteria for BPD than were those without such evidence (P = .0016). In addition, patients reporting childhood sexual abuse were 2.9 times more likely to have met criteria for BPD than those who did not report being sexually abused before the age of 18 (P = .0410).

DISCUSSION

Our study examined 1) whether borderline patients (or a subset of borderline patients) have developmental or acquired CNS dysfunction that distinguishes them from control subjects with

Table 9–2. Prevalence of pathological childhood experiences in borderline patients with and without vulnerable CNS substrate

Experience	% BPD with vulnerable CNS substrate	% BPD without vulnerable CNS substrate
Verbal abuse*	80.0	20.0
Emotional abuse	82.9	80.0
Physical abuse	60.0	20.0
Sexual abuse	74.3	100.0
Physical neglect	40.0	0.0
Emotional withdrawal	71.4	40.0
Inconsistent treatment by caretaker	60.0	40.0
Emotional denial by caretaker	80.0	60.0
No real relationship with caretaker	77.1	80.0
Parentification of patient by caretaker	74.3	60.0
Failure to protect by caretaker	65.7	60.0
Caretaker malevolence	68.6	20.0

Note. BPD = borderline personality disorder. CNS = central nervous system.
*Significant at P < .05.

personality disorders and 2) whether pathological childhood experiences such as abuse and neglect would be significantly related to neurological dysfunction or "vulnerability." Three main findings emerged from our study. First, borderline patients had a relatively high incidence of maternal drug or alcohol use, complications of birth or pregnancy, developmental reading or writing impairments, arithmetic impairments, and a history of head injuries. However, none of these variables significantly discriminated borderline patients from control subjects with personality disorders. Second, borderline patients were significantly more likely than control subjects with personality disorders to have evidence for some sort of neurological vulnerability. Third, a "vulnerable neurological substrate" was a stronger predictor of BPD than was a reported childhood history of sexual abuse.

Incidence of Neurological Dysfunction

Our study sought to examine the prevalence of neurodevelopmental and acquired CNS dysfunction in borderline patients. Our findings of 22.5% reported developmental reading impairment, 40% reported developmental arithmetic impairment, and 12.5% reported childhood ADHD are consistent with Andrulonis' finding of between 40% and 52% prevalence of ADHD and/or learning disability. Our most striking neurodevelopmental finding was the reported incidence of 32.5% developmental speech and language delays. This was significantly greater than Soloff and Millward (1983), who found only one to two patients in each group with reported speech and language difficulty. We also found more reported complications of birth and pregnancy (32.5%) than Soloff and Millward (17.8%). These findings may not be inconsistent, however, because we combined reports of complications of pregnancy, complications of birth, and prematurity, whereas Soloff and Millward reported them separately, and it is unclear how many different patients their three variables represent.

It is notable that 87.5% of our borderline patients demonstrated some form of brain injury when these factors were considered: maternal alcohol and drug exposure, speech and language difficulty, head injury history (including drug and alcohol blackouts), seizure history, and a diagnosis of ADHD. Our results are consistent with Andrulonis and colleagues' organic subgroup of borderline patients (Andrulonis and Vogel 1984; Andrulonis et al. 1981, 1982). Andrulonis' patients with a history of "organicity" had ADHD or a learning disability and/or acquired brain trauma, encephalitis, or epilepsy. Our results are also consistent with the finding by Van Reekum et al. (1993) that a large proportion (81%) of borderline patients may have some form of brain injury.

In our study, having at least one neurological finding thought to represent probable vulnerable CNS substrate was found to discriminate BPD from other Axis II disorders with high significance. However, none of the individual variables was significantly more frequent in borderline subjects than in control subjects with personality disorders. This suggests that neurological vulnerabilities are common but nondiscriminating among patients with personality disorders. It also suggests that there is no single CNS dysfunction specifically related to BPD, but rather that having some nonspecific form of CNS dysfunction may be relevant to BPD.

Comparison With Previous Literature

Our conclusion that there is evidence for brain dysfunction as a relevant risk factor for BPD is consistent with the conclusions of Andrulonis and colleagues and Van Reekum and colleagues; it differs from that of Soloff and Millward (1983) and this group's later review by Cornelius et al. (1989), which concluded that their findings did not suggest a significant role for neurodevelopmental deficits and suggested that organic developmental factors are unlikely or uncommon as risk factors for BPD.

Our findings suggest that patients with some form of neurological dysfunction are 6 times more likely to be borderline than patients without some form of neurological dysfunction. In our sample, having some form of neurological dysfunction was a stronger predictor of BPD than was childhood sexual abuse. This finding suggests that having some form of neurological dysfunction, either developmental or acquired, may be a factor more relevant to the development of BPD than is a childhood history of sexual abuse. It must be noted that our work does not discriminate between developmental and acquired dysfunction, because many of the variables studied may be secondary to both developmental and acquired injury. It is possible that sexual abuse itself (or the environment in which it occurs) leads to subtle neurological impairment or vulnerability (e.g., arrested maturation, learning difficulties, more frequent head injuries, seizure, or seizurelike disorders).

Although Soloff and Millward's results appear to contradict the arguments proposed by Andrulonis and coauthors and supported in our study, it should be noted that by excluding patients with organic and substance abuse problems, Soloff and Millward excluded many subjects who were the type of borderline patient described by Andrulonis's group and by our group. Although substance abuse, particularly alcohol abuse, is very common among borderline patients (Zanarini et al. 1989a), it is also very relevant to any consideration of an organic substrate (Oepen et al. 1993).

Furthermore, the studies discussed above that found significant evidence for organicity in BPD (Andrulonis and Vogel 1984; Andrulonis et al. 1981, 1982; Van Reekum et al. 1993) included mostly male subjects, whereas Soloff and Millward's sample had 84.4% female patients, and our own sample consists exclusively of female patients. This is highly relevant, because organic impairment in general seems to be more prevalent among males. We might expect, therefore, to see even more organic pathology in our male study participants. In addition, Soloff and Millward (1983) compared BPD patients with control subjects who had schizophrenia and depression. Given that neurological abnormalities have been demonstrated in schizophrenia (Woods et al. 1986), the usefulness of this comparison is not clear.

Role of CNS Dysfunction in BPD

If CNS injury is relevant to BPD, two aspects seem of particular importance: 1) timing of a hypothetical CNS injury and 2) specificity of the dysfunction, with differing effects on resulting psychopathology. As to timing, both prenatal drug exposure and childhood speech and language disorder might suggest neurological dysfunction developing in utero or in early development, suggestive of a neurological predisposition (or "vulnerability") to later developed psychopathology. This can be seen in support of CNS dysfunction at a critical and early time of brain (and personality) development, in utero or in early childhood, as a relevant factor for the later diagnosis of BPD. In a developmental neuropsychological model, this might provide the framework to explain developmental delays, failed maturation, and integration of higher cerebral functions, along with consequent problems in areas such as identity, memory, and affect regulation (Gazzaniga and LeDoux 1978). In earlier research on MBD (Rutter 1982), the possibility of diffuse versus specific localizing brain dysfunction (mostly frontal lobe), and its possible role in later psychopathology, was raised. Neither MBD nor any other concept of neurological dysfunction affecting behavior can realistically be evaluated outside a social and dynamic context; therefore, none of these factors can ever alone be predictive of psychopathology.

Similar concerns hold true for specificity. It is notable that none of the items indicative of posterior CNS dysfunction, such as developmental reading and writing disorder or developmental arithmetic disorder, was significant, in contrast to a trend toward significance for "childhood speech and language disorder," which might suggest evidence for some localizing specificity (anterior and left brain regions). Given that estimates of the prevalence of language disorders in the general population range from 1% to 21% for developmental articulation disorder (Cantwell and Baker 1987), the 32.5% prevalence in our borderline sample is a notable finding. This can be compared with the finding by Teicher et al. (1994) of a correlation between abuse and EEG abnormalities predominantly in the left frontal region in adolescents. One could speculate about the significance of the left anterior hemisphere for expressive language functions, dysarthria, and depersonalization, as well as the possible role of (mainly left-hemispheric) language-based processes and their impairment for communication, and presumably, then, the later development of defense mechanisms, ego functions, and identity (Oepen et al. 1988). On the other hand, the argument for specific left anterior brain dysfunction in BPD is not supported;

rather, there is a greater predictive value of nonspecific CNS dysfunction. This is further underlined by the higher prevalence of ADHD and fine motor incoordination in our BPD group, which may be seen as indicative of frontal lobe dysfunction, but without any specific laterality. In summary, our preliminary data suggest but do not support any specific localized brain dysfunction in BPD. Alternatively, our results can be considered as indicative of and consistent with psychosocial models of borderline personality. Psychodynamic models of BPD have postulated that BPD represents complex characterological difficulties relating to ego development as it occurs in the patient's childhood environment. Our finding of high rates of maternal drug and alcohol abuse in both borderline subjects and control subjects with personality disorders may indicate the presence of an emotionally impaired caregiver, whose effect on the developing child might be as significant as, or more significant than, the effects of in utero exposure to drugs or alcohol. An emotionally impoverished childhood environment could contribute to speech or language delay in borderline patients. McCormack (1991) noted that developmental delay resulting from sexual abuse may inadvertently be labeled learning disability. It is highly possible that much of the neurological dysfunction in our sample is directly related to a neglectful or abusive environment. However, it is worth noting that in our previous retrospective study (Zanarini et al. 1994), physical abuse was not correlated with reported head injury or seizure disorders, variables studied to reflect neurological dysfunction.

Pathological Childhood Experiences

Our hypothesis was that pathological childhood experiences might in some way interact with neurological abnormalities in borderline patients. Based on a substantial literature documenting increased risk of childhood abuse and neglect in borderline patients (see Zanarini, Chapter 1, this volume), for a review of the relevant studies), we expected to find high rates of both childhood abuse and childhood neglect. Although we found these high rates of abuse and neglect, no specific pathological childhood experience was reported significantly more frequently by our borderline patients than by patients with other personality disorders. This finding is not unexpected, given the severity of illness currently required for inpatient hospitalization.

When each childhood variable could be considered independently in the logistic regression, with other variables held constant, sexual abuse was the only childhood experience that significantly predicted BPD. Although there was not a significant difference between patients with and without vulnerable CNS substrate with regard to sexual abuse, 100% of the patients without a vulnerable CNS substrate reported a childhood history of sexual abuse. This might suggest that 1) there are different "pathways" to developing borderline personality and 2) when neurological vulnerability is not present, sexual abuse is a critical etiological factor. This hypothesis would need to be tested in a larger sample. It is likely, however, that the etiology of borderline personality remains a complex interaction of both biological and environmental factors.

How can we understand the interaction of abuse and neurological vulnerability in BPD? First, these two risk factors could occur independently and, in comorbid individuals, could create a high risk for BPD. Second, as proposed by van der Kolk and Greenberg (1987) and by Teicher et al. (1994), traumatic childhood experiences could have neurobiological consequences, or, in parallel, interfere with neurological development as well as with psychological development and thus lead to impaired personality development. Third, neurological vulnerability might in some way single out children, rendering them at greater risk of being abused (Davies 1979), which in turn could lead to impaired personality development. Fourth, pathological childhood experiences and neurological vulnerability could define two separate borderline subpopulations. Patients may develop BPD through a pathway of abuse and neglect or through a pathway of neurological injury, and the two subgroups may be situated on a continuum or spectrum of psychopathology, with differences in symptoms, comorbidity, treatment response, and lifetime course and outcome. Our data are consistent with each of these models but do not allow us any definitive conclusions. Determining which of these models holds true awaits prospective longitudinal studies of high-risk children.

Limitations and Conclusions

Our study is limited by its relatively small sample size, which may not have given us sufficient power to find significant between-group differences. In addition, using patient self-reports in a retrospective design without using independent confirmation may yield inaccuracies, although this bias should be equal for both borderline and control patients.

Avenues we plan to explore include symptoms of temporal lobe epilepsy, EEG results, and evidence for hormonal or endocrinological dysregulation. We also plan to explore the relationship between these types of neurological dysfunction and 1) the severity of substance abuse (in analogy to Oepen et al. 1993) and 2) the severity of pathological childhood experiences.

Finally, several interesting questions arise. Is there a relationship between certain forms of organic impairment, certain childhood experiences, and specific psychopathological symptoms? Do neurologically vulnerable borderline patients have clinical traits different from those of borderline patients without such vulnerability, such as being more impulsive or self-destructive? Do borderline patients with evidence for neurological dysfunction respond differently to medication than those without such evidence? Will borderline patients with neurological dysfunction have a poorer outcome when followed longitudinally? These questions await long-term prospective follow-up. We are currently engaged in such a study, which we hope will shed more light on the role of developmental or acquired neurological dysfunction and its interaction with pathological childhood experiences in the etiology of BPD.

REFERENCES

American Psychiatric Association: Diagnostic and Statistical Manual of Mental Disorders, 3rd Edition. Washington, DC, American Psychiatric Association, 1980

American Psychiatric Association: Diagnostic and Statistical Manual of Mental Disorders, 3rd Edition, Revised. Washington, DC, American Psychiatric Association, 1987

Andrulonis PA, Vogel NG: Comparison of borderline personality sub-categories to schizophrenic and affective disorders. Br J Psychiatry 144:358–363, 1984

Andrulonis PA, Glueck BC, Stroebel CF, et al: Organic brain dysfunction and the borderline syndrome. Psychiatr Clin North Am 4:47–66, 1981

Andrulonis PA, Glueck BC, Stroebel CF, et al: Borderline personality subcategories. J Nerv Ment Dis 170:670–679, 1982

Cantwell PC, Baker L: Developmental Speech and Language Disorders. New York, Guilford Press, 1987

Cornelius JR, Soloff PH, George AWA, et al: An evaluation of the significance of selected neuropsychiatric abnormalities in the etiology of BPD. Journal of Personality Disorders 3:19–25, 1989

Davies RK: Incest: some neuropsychiatric findings. Int J Psychiatry Med 9:117–121, 1979

Fyer MR, Frances AJ, Sullivan T, et al: Comorbidity of BPD. Arch Gen Psychiatry 45:348–352, 1988

Gazzaniga MS, LeDoux JE: The Integrated Mind. New York, Plenum, 1978

Herman JL, Perry JC, van der Kolk BA: Childhood trauma in BPD. Am J Psychiatry 146:490–495, 1989

Links PS, Steiner M, Offord DR, et al: Characteristics of BPD: a Canadian study. Can J Psychiatry 33:336–340, 1988

McCormack B: Sexual abuse and learning disabilities. Br Med J 303:143–144, 1991

Oepen G, Harrington A, Spitzer M, et al: "Feelings" of conviction—on the relation of affect and thought disorder, in Psychopathology and Philosophy. Edited by Spitzer M, Uehlein FA, Oepen G. New York, Springer-Verlag, 1988, pp 43–55

Oepen G, Levy M, Saemann R, et al: A neuropsychological perspective on dual diagnosis: a Jacksonian model. J Psychoactive Drugs 252:129–133, 1993

Ogata SN, Silk KR, Goodrich S, et al: Childhood sexual and physical abuse in adult patients with BPD. Am J Psychiatry 147:1008–1013, 1990

Rutter M: Syndromes attributed to "minimal brain dysfunction" in childhood. Am J Psychiatry 139:21–33, 1982

Shearer SL, Peters CP, Quaytman MS, et al: Frequency and correlates of childhood sexual and physical abuse histories in adult female borderline inpatients. Am J Psychiatry 147:214–216, 1990

Soloff PH, Millward JW: Developmental histories of borderline patients. Compr Psychiatry 24:574–588, 1983

Teicher MH, Ito Y, Glod CA, et al: Early abuse, limbic system dysfunction, and BPD, in Biological and Neurobehavioral Studies of Borderline Personality Disorder. Edited by Silk KR. Washington, DC, American Psychiatric Press, 1994, pp 177–207 van der Kolk BA, Greenberg MS: The psychobiology of the trauma response: developmental issues in the psychobiology of attachment and separation, in Psychological Trauma. Edited by van der Kolk BA. Washington, DC, American Psychiatric Press, 1987, pp 63–87

Van Reekum R, Conway CA, Gansler D, et al: Neurobehavioral study of BPD. J Psychiatry Neurosci 18:121–129, 1993

Westen D, Ludolph P, Misle B, et al: Physical and sexual abuse in adolescent girls with BPD. Am J Orthopsychiatry 60:55–66, 1990

Woods BT, Kinney DK, Yurgelun-Todd D: Neurological abnormalities in schizophrenic patients and their families. Arch Gen Psychiatry 43:657–663, 1986

Zanarini MC, Gunderson JG, Frankenburg FR: Axis I phenomenology of BPD. Compr Psychiatry 30:149–156, 1989a

Zanarini MC, Gunderson JG, Marino MF, et al: Childhood experiences of borderline patients. Compr Psychiatry 30:18–25, 1989b

Zanarini MC, Kimble CR, Williams AA: Neurological dysfunction in borderline patients and Axis II control subjects, in Biological and Neurobehavioral Studies of Borderline Personality Disorder. Edited by Silk KR. Washington, DC, American Psychiatric Press, 1994, pp 159–175

Chapter 10

A History of Childhood Sexual Abuse and the Course of Borderline Personality Disorder

M. Janice E. Mitton, R.N., B.A., M.H.Sc.,
Paul S. Links, M.D., F.R.C.P.(C.), M.Sc., and
Gerald Durocher, B.A., M.A.

Recent reports in the literature provide a growing body of evidence that childhood abuse (including childhood sexual abuse [CSA], physical abuse, early separation or loss, biparental failure, and abnormal parental bonding) is a significant factor in the development of borderline psychopathology (Links et al. 1990b).

More specifically, a history of CSA has been shown in one independent study to be the most significant abuse variable in female inpatients who met criteria for borderline personality disorder (BPD) (Paris et al. 1993). One of the authors of this chapter reported (Links and van Reekum 1993) that a history of CSA made an independent contribution to the level of borderline psychopathology after the effects of other types of abuse or disadvantage were controlled for.

Other clinicians and researchers have chronicled the long-term aftereffects of CSA. Many of the most frequently reported of these aftereffects (symptoms of depression and/or anxiety, poor self-esteem, suicidal and self-destructive tendencies, substance abuse, relationship problems, dissociative experiences, symptoms of posttraumatic stress disorder, and sexual dysfunction) are also common in BPD (Beitchman et al. 1992; Briere 1992; Browne and Finkelhor 1986; Herman 1992; Schetky 1990; Sheldrick 1991; Starr et al. 1991).

From these observations, CSA is now considered an important risk factor in the development of BPD. The impact of a history of CSA in follow-up studies, however, has not been routinely examined as a prognostic factor explaining course and outcome for the borderline diagnosis. In this chapter we review the recent literature with this purpose in mind and present data on CSA as a prognostic factor from a recently completed prospective 7-year follow-up study of formerly hospitalized borderline patients. The implications of these findings for clinical practice and future research are discussed.

Specifically, we examine the relationship between a reported history of CSA and three outcome categories: 1) perpetuation of the BPD diagnosis and of borderline symptomatology, 2) other parameters of psychiatric illness (e.g., symptoms or diagnoses along Axes I and II, number of psychiatric rehospitalizations, time spent in psychiatric facilities), and 3) long-term social and occupational functioning.

BACKGROUND

Generally, studies examining long-term outcome in BPD reported improvement after 15 years' follow-up; half of the BPD patients were considered "recovered" at 15-year follow-up, a minority of subjects did poorly, and suicide rates varied from approximately 3% to 10% (McGlashan 1986; Paris et al. 1987; Plakun et al. 1985; Stone 1991).

To examine outcome at 7-year follow-up for BPD subjects who reported a history of CSA, we undertook a review of the literature. To our knowledge, only one study (Stone 1991) has examined the relationship between BPD, CSA, and long-term outcome. Stone's sample was drawn from a population of adolescent and young adult patients admitted for at least 3 months to a unit specializing in intensive psychoanalytically oriented psychotherapy at the New York State Psychiatric Institute. Stone compared 28 female and 7 male former inpatients who had BPD by DSM-III criteria (American Psychiatric Association 1980) and who also had a history of incest with the remainder of those in his sample.

Subjects were identified by a retrospective chart review, using a checklist of borderline criteria from DSM-III-R. Follow-up assessment was done with a semistructured clinical interview that inquired about rehospitalization, subsequent therapy, work history, social network, avocational interests, marriage, and child rearing. Most (93%) of the interviews were done by phone. Stone found a significant difference in the distribution of abused and nonabused female borderline patients when the Global Assessment Scale (GAS) outcome score was dichotomized into Well versus Unwell. There were no differences in suicide rates between the two groups (3/28 [11%] for the abused group vs. 8/116 [7%] for the nonabused group). Of 7 male BPD+CSA subjects, 2 completed suicide, and the mean GAS score for the remaining 5 was 80.5, suggesting a greater variability in the outcomes of male than of female borderline patients with a childhood history of abuse.

CURRENT STUDY

The current study offers several advantages over earlier follow-up studies, which were "catch-up" studies of borderline subjects. First, the current study is a real-time prospective follow-up of the same cohort of borderline subjects. In contrast, most of the earlier studies were retrospective studies, in which adequacy and accuracy of the initial records were not ensured. Second, the current methodology employed direct assessment of both Axes I and II via valid, reliable instruments. Third, repeated examination of the same cohort of subjects was made, which may provide insight into the mechanisms of change in a borderline population reporting a history of CSA.

Subjects

Subjects were derived from an ongoing prospective follow-up study of BPD and many (at time of publication of this volume) have been assessed at three points in time (intake and two follow-up points). At initial intake (time 1), subjects were inpatients between the ages of 18 and 65 in one of four acute psychiatric care settings associated with McMaster University, Faculty of Health Sciences, Department of Psychiatry, Hamilton, Ontario, Canada. Referral was based on a suspected clinical diagnosis of BPD. Exclusion criteria included a diagnosis of organic brain disorder, epilepsy, IQ below 80, and inability to understand English. For purposes of the study, the diagnosis of BPD was made by using the Diagnostic Interview for Borderlines (DIB) (Gunderson et al. 1981). Axis I was assessed with the Schedule for Affective Disorders and Schizophrenia, both Current and Lifetime versions (SADS) (Endicott and Spitzer 1978). Diagnoses were made according to Research Diagnostic Criteria (RDC) (Spitzer et al. 1978). The Childhood Antecedents Questionnaire (CAQ), a 24-item, interviewer-scored checklist of childhood loss events, abuse, and antisocial behaviors, was used at time 1 to assess physical and sexual abuse (Reitsma-Street et al. 1985). All available sources of data regarding abuse were used to score the CAQ. Because the CAQ was not systematized, one of us (M.J.M.) developed the following definition of CSA for use with the questionnaire: either a single, traumatic incident (e.g., rape) or any kind of repetitive sexual abuse involving physical contact. In addition, perpetrators had to have had a caregiving role with the subject at the time of the abuse. More detail regarding methodology at time 1 is reported elsewhere (Links et al. 1988).

Of 130 subjects referred at time 1, 88 met DIB criteria for BPD. These 88 subjects were reassessed at 2 years after index contact (time 2) (mean follow-up = 19.3 months; range = 7–28 months). Methodology for time 2 is also reported elsewhere (Links et al. 1990a). An attempt was made to reassess all 126 survivors from time 1 at 5- to 7-year follow-up (time 3) (mean follow-up = 81.4 months; range = 67–103 months). The rater was blind to all data from times 1 and 2.

Subjects at Time 3

At time 3, two subgroups were drawn from the original cohort of 88 patients who met DIB criteria at time 1 for a diagnosis of BPD. Twenty-two of these 88 patients reported a history of CSA. They are referred to here as the *abused group* for purposes of this chapter. Of these 22 abused subjects, we were able to reassess 14 at time 3.

The 14 abused subjects were matched to 14 subjects who also had BPD at time 1 but who did not report a history of CSA. For the rest of the chapter, this control or matched-pairs group will be referred to as the *nonabused group.*

In addition to meeting DIB criteria for BPD, the two groups were also matched on the following variables: age ± 4 years (mean age of the abused group at time 1 was 25.1 years [SD = 6.2] and 26.1 years for the nonabused group [SD = 6.8]), gender (13 female, 1 male), and a score of ± 10 on the Peabody Picture Vocabulary Test (PPVT) (Dunn and Dunn 1981).

When the abused and nonabused borderline groups were compared on initial variables, they differed significantly on only one variable: mean age at which they first sought outpatient psychiatric care (13.1 years for the abused group vs. 18.9 years for the nonabused group, $t = -3.65$, df = 13, $P = .003$). To further assess confounding variables, the two groups were compared on the CAQ. A principal-components factor analysis (with oblique rotation) of the CAQ items was carried out on the original sample of 130 subjects. Factors having eigenvalues greater than 1 were retained, which resulted in the following factors: Delinquent Behavior ($\alpha = .85$); Separation from Caretaker ($\alpha = .64$); School Failure ($\alpha = .70$); and Violent Behavior ($\alpha = .66$). Of these, only School Failure correlated significantly with a history of childhood sexual abuse ($r = .57$, $n = 27$, $P < .001$).

The abused borderline patients also had higher scores at time 1 on individual DIB items measuring a pattern of substance abuse, derealization, and depersonalization; on three DIB section scores (Impulse Action Patterns, Psychosis, and Interpersonal Relationships), and on the Total DIB section score.

Lost to Follow-Up

Of the original 22 BPD subjects who reported a history of CSA at time 1, 8 were lost to follow-up at time 3 for the following reasons: 1 suicide, 5 refusals, and 2 not located. To ensure that a selection bias did not exist for those lost to follow-up, they were compared to the followed abused group on the time 1 variables of age, sex, score on the PPVT, total number of psychiatric hospitalizations, age at which they first sought outpatient psychiatric services, and the section and scaled section scores of the DIB. No significant differences were found.

Follow-Up Methods

Measures used at follow-up included the following seven instruments:

1. *The Schedule for Affective Disorders and Schizophrenia—Lifetime Interval Version (SADS-LI).* The SADS-LI (Spitzer and Endicott 1984) covered the period from the subject's most recent interview up to the time of the current interview and was used to assess Axis I disorders for a specified period.
2. *Research Diagnostic Criteria—Third Edition and Third Edition Updated (RDC).* The RDC (Spitzer et al. 1978, 1989) were used to determine episodes of mental illness.
3. *McGlashan Outcome Dimensions.* This 5-point, interviewer-rated scale was used to assess five areas of functioning over the entire period of follow-up: percentage of time spent in a psychiatric facility, employment, social activity, psychopathology, and global functioning. The scale covers the entire period of follow-up being assessed. As the score increases, from 0 to 4, so does functioning (McGlashan 1984).
4. *DIB.* The original version of the DIB (Gunderson et al. 1981) was used to assess the presence or absence of borderline psychopathology and the borderline diagnosis at times 2 and 3. At time 3, the DIB was used in combination with its revised version, the DIB-R (Zanarini et al. 1989), which has been found to be more specific to borderline than to other personality disorders.
5. *Structured Interview for DSM-III-R Personality Disorders (SIDP-R).* The SIDP-R (Pfohl et al. 1989) was used to assess conditions along Axis II. This semistructured interview consists of 159 questions arranged in topical sections. A subset of questions is asked of an informant who knows the subject well. All information is then used to determine the presence or absence

of diagnostic criteria for the 13 categories of personality disorders by DSM-III-R criteria, including BPD.

6. *Suicidal Behaviors Questionnaire (SBQ).* The SBQ inquires about the subject's self-harm and suicidal ideation within the previous 6 months and into the future (Linehan 1983).

7. *Social Adjustment Scale—Self-Report (SAS-SR).* The SAS-SR measures social and leisure activities, relationship with extended family, marital role, parental role, family unity, and economic independence. The period is the previous 2 weeks (Weissman and Bothwell 1976; Weissman et al. 1978). Adaptive functioning on the SAS-SR has been shown to be a reliable predictor of good prognosis in psychiatric inpatients (Mellsop et al. 1987).

Data Analysis

To examine the effect over time that reporting a history of CSA might have on a patient with a diagnosis of BPD, results were compared between the matched pairs of subjects on variables measuring the three categories of outcome described above.

A repeated-measures analysis of variance (ANOVA) was employed separately on each outcome variable, using a 2-factor (2 × 3) repeated measures design. Two within-subject variables were involved: the first was CSA (presence or absence of) and the second was time (i.e., baseline and the two follow-up periods). Because of the sample sizes involved and the preliminary nature of the results, interpretation of results was done without consideration of the Bonferroni correction for multiple univariate comparisons. (Variables that meet the probability levels associated with the Bonferroni correction for multiple univariate comparisons are noted in Tables 10–1 through 10–4.)

Results Over Time

A similar and significant pattern of improvement over time was found for both groups of subjects—that is, a change in the same direction was noted for both the abused and the nonabused borderline patients. These improvements are summarized in the following paragraphs with respect to the three outcome categories studied, noted in the first part of the chapter.

Perpetuation of BPD Symptomatology

As Table 10–1 shows, both groups showed an improvement over time alone on all eight DSM-III-R criteria for BPD ($P < .05$ for criterion 5, affective instability; $P < .001$ for all other criteria).

As Table 10–2 shows, similar improvement was also noted on the following individual items from the DIB: active social life (Social Activities); conventional appearance (Appearance/Manners) ($P < . 05$); suicidal threats, attempts, or gestures (Manipulative Suicide); pattern of substance abuse (Drug Abuse) ($P = .001$); recent or chronic symptoms of clinical depression (Depression); chronic dysphoria, or anhedonia (Dysphoria/Anhedonia) ($P = .001$); angry affect (Hostility) ($P = .05$); Derealization ($P = .05$); drug-free psychotic depressed experiences (Depressive) ($P = .001$); and problems with manipulation, hostility, or devaluation in close relationships (Devaluation/Manipulation) ($P < .05$).

Both groups also showed significant improvements in the section and scaled section scores on three of the five sections of the DIB: Social Adaptation ($P < .05$), Impulse Action Patterns ($P < .001$), and Affects ($P < .004$), as well as the total section and scaled section DIB scores.

This within-group pattern of improvement over time was also noted on the SADS item that measures total number of suicidal gestures or attempts ($P = .007$).

Other Parameters of Psychiatric Illness

Improvement for both groups over time was found on two items from the SADS, number of psychiatric hospitalizations ($P = .012$) and total time spent in a psychiatric hospital ($P = .042$), and on McGlashan's follow-up measure of psychopathology ($P = .001$).

Table 10–1. Mean scores on individual DSM-III-R criteria

Criterion	Time 1		Time 2		Time 3		P values[a]		
	CSA	Non-CSA	CSA	Non-CSA	CSA	Non-CSA	Time	CSA	CSA × time
Impulsivity, unpredictability	1.9	1.7	1.9	1.6	1.3	0.8	.000	.148	.666
Unstable, intense relationship	1.9	1.6	1.6	1.2	0.9	0.4	.000[b]	.051	.946
Inappropriate intense anger	1.7	1.7	1.9	1.4	1.0	1.0	.001[b]	.167	.085
Identity disturbance[c]	1.5	1.5	1.5	1.2	0.9	0.5	.000[b]	.146	.416
Affective instability[c]	1.7	1.4	1.6	1.5	1.7	0.6	.014	.009	.004
Intolerance of being alone	1.9	1.4	1.6	1.5	0.3	0.0	.000[b]	.054	.232
Self-damaging acts	2.0	1.8	1.6	1.5	1.4	1.0	.000[b]	.208	.769
Chronic feelings of emptiness, boredom	1.9	1.8	1.6	1.5	0.7	0.1	.000[b]	.070	.098

[a]From analysis of variance for time alone; $P < .05$ for affective instability, $P < .001$ for all other criteria listed.
[b]Statistically significant according to Bonferroni's correction for multiple comparisons.

Table 10–2. Mean scores on DIB items and section scores

Feature description	Time 1		Time 2		Time 3		P values[a]		
	CSA	Non-CSA	CSA	Non-CSA	CSA	Non-CSA	Time	CSA	CSA × time
Social adaptation									
School/work achievement	1.7	1.4	1.5	1.2	1.5	1.0	.352	.079	.762
Special abilities/talent	1.0	1.2	1.1	1.2	1.2	1.3	.792	.441	.978
Social activities	0.8	0.5	0.8	1.4	1.2	1.4	.015	.502	.123
Appearance/manners	1.6	1.8	1.4	1.9	2.0	2.0	.015	.095	.097
Section score	4.7	4.9	4.8	5.7	5.9	5.7	.025	.447	.279
Scaled section score	1.8	2.0	1.7	1.8	2.0	2.0	.012	.165	.467
Impulse action patterns									
Self-mutilation	1.6	1.2	1.1	0.8	1.2	0.4	.115	.004	.330
Manipulative suicide	1.7	1.7	1.5	1.2	1.2	0.7	.002	.254	.457
Drug abuse	1.5	0.8	1.0	0.8	0.7	0.2	.002	.163	.290
Sexual deviance	0.8	0.3	0.4	0.5	0.6	0.5	.845	.552	.410
Antisocial	1.5	1.2	1.3	1.2	1.4	0.8	.625[b]	.139	.744
Section score	7.0	5.2	5.2	4.3	5.1	2.6	.000[b]	.015	.356
Scaled section score	1.8	1.4	1.4	1.0	1.3	0.6	.001[b]	.018	.411
Affects									
Depression	1.9	1.9	1.5	1.8	1.6	0.8	.001[b]	.366	.006
Hostility	1.8	1.5	1.7	0.7	1.5	0.7	.023	.004	.053
Demanding/entitled	1.2	1.0	0.8	0.5	1.0	0.7	.211[b]	.146	.902
Dysphoria/anhedonia	1.8	2.0	1.5	1.3	1.5	0.8	.001[b]	.373	.009
Flat/elated (-)[c]	0.1	0.2	0.0	0.1	0.1	0.0	.037	.502	.433
Section score	6.6	6.2	5.5	4.3	5.5	2.9	.005	.011	.066
Scaled section score	2.0	1.8	1.5	1.4	1.7	0.8	.004	.033	.074

Psychosis									
Derealization	1.2	0.7	0.6	0.3	1.1	0.1	.051	.026	.232
Depersonalization	1.2	0.6	1.0	0.4	0.7	0.2	.189	.020	.941
Depressive	1.2	1.2	0.8	0.6	0.9	0.4	.003	.119[b]	.176
Paranoid	0.8	0.3	1.0	0.3	1.1	0.3	.732	.001[b]	.788
Drug-induced	0.2	0.0	0.2	0.3	0.4	0.2	.273	.746	.546
Hallucinations (-)[c]	0.2	0.0	0.3	0.0	0.4	0.1	.069	.190	.167
Mania (-)[c]	0.2	0.0	0.1	0.2	0.3	0.2	.027	.730	.695
Therapy regressions	1.1	0.8	1.4	1.0	0.6	0.7	.055	.512	.540
Section score	5.2	3.5	4.7	2.7	4.0	1.9	.068	.012	.932
Scaled section score$_r$	1.5	1.2	1.5	1.1	1.5	0.7	.295	.054	.464
Interpersonal features									
Aloneness	1.5	0.7	0.8	1.0	1.2	0.7	.759	.110	.032[a]
Isolation (-)[c]	0.2	0.7	0.1	0.0	0.3	0.1	.003	.006	.383
Anaclitic	1.1	1.0	1.2	1.0	1.5	1.0	.478	.352	.418
Instability	0.8	0.8	1.0	0.7	0.9	0.8	.980	.441	.897
Devaluation/manipulation	1.2	1.2	0.9	0.5	0.6	0.5	.016	.292	.535
Dependency/masochism	1.5	1.4	1.3	1.0	1.0	0.8	.107	.386	.894
Past-therapy relations	1.1	1.3	1.4	0.8	0.8	0.7	.056	.517	.027
Section score	7.0	5.7	6.2	4.9	5.8	6.2	.734	.504	.473
Scaled section score	1.8	1.5	1.6	1.2	1.5	1.2	.149	.118	.928
Total section scores	31.4	25.3	27.3	21.0	26.6	17.3	.004	.005	.429
Total scaled section scores	9.0	7.9	7.6	6.5	7.9	5.3	.002	.028	.087

[a] From analysis of variance.
[b] Statistically significant according to Bonferroni's correction for multiple comparisons.
[c] (-) indicates not typical of borderline patients.

Social and Occupational Functioning

Significant within-group improvement over time was noted on two of McGlashan's follow-up measures: employment ($P = .025$) and global functioning ($P = .001$).

Results: Time Plus Childhood Sexual Abuse

The interaction of BPD and CSA over time gives a more complete picture of long-term functioning for the abused group. Results are again presented in the three categories studied.

Perpetuation of BPD Diagnosis

To examine perpetuation of BPD diagnosis in relation to CSA, various classification schemes for borderline patients were compared across time. At time 3, 93% of the abused borderline subjects, compared to 54% of the nonabused borderline subjects, continued to meet DSM-III-R criteria for a diagnosis of BPD ($t = 2.58$, df $= 13$, $P = .023$).

No differentiation between abused and nonabused subjects across time or at time 3 was evident for the DIB or DIB-R criteria.

Perpetuation of BPD Symptomatology

As Table 10–1 shows, all eight DSM-III-R criteria for BPD were examined across time with respect to CSA. Only Affective Instability showed a time × CSA interaction ($F = 7.2$, df $= 2/12$, $P < .01$): the nonabused group showed more improvement than did the abused group. Examination of mean scores shows that this change was most prominent from time 2 to time 3 and that the abused group remained virtually the same on this item across all three points in time.

Section scores, scaled section scores, and individual items were examined on the DIB across time. As Table 10–2 shows, no scaled section or section scores were found to differentiate CSA over time. Two items each, however, in the affects and in the interpersonal relationships sections did show a difference. They were recent/chronic symptoms of clinical depression and chronic dysphoria or anhedonia, for which the nonabused group showed improvement over time, most notably from time 2 to time 3; tries to avoid being alone, on which the abused group initially showed a decrease from time 1 to time 2 and then an increase at time 3; and staff splitting/countertransference problems, for which the nonabused group showed a decline across both follow-up periods, whereas the abused group demonstrated a large increase at time 2 followed by a decrease at time 3. Comparisons of the DIB-R were made by using Student's *t* test, because that measure was given at time 3 only. Results from this analysis (Table 10–3) showed that although the DIB-R did not differentiate the two groups for a diagnosis of BPD, the abused group had greater DIB-R scores in several categories.

The abused group scored higher on 5 of the 22 individual summary statements: sustained feelings of helplessness; frequent symptoms of anxiety; transient, nondelusional paranoid experiences; a pattern of physical self-mutilation; and strong counterdependence in interpersonal relationships. In addition, in terms of inspection of means for trend, almost all other individual DIB-R item scores were higher for the abused group.

The section and scaled section scores from the areas of affect, cognition, and impulse action patterns were all statistically higher at time 3 for the abused group. Only the section score measuring interpersonal relationships did not show a difference. The abused group also scored higher on the total DIB-R score.

Suicidal Behaviors Questionnaire

As Table 10–4 shows, the abused group scored higher than the nonabused group on two items from the SBQ at time 3: How often have you thought about hurting yourself? and Chances of hurting yourself within the next 6 months.

Other Parameters of Psychiatric Illness

The two groups were compared on all Axis I lifetime diagnoses rated by the SADS. Because of small numbers in many categories, diagnoses were compared individually and then collapsed

Table 10–3.   Mean scores on DIB-R items and section scores at time 3

Feature	CSA	Non-CSA	P values[a]
Affective features			
Chronic/major depression	1.6	1.2	.355
Chronic feelings of helplessness	1.6	1.0	.045
Chronic anger/frequent angry acts	1.5	1.1	.174
Chronic anxiety	1.6	0.7	.017
Chronic loneliness/boredom/emptiness	1.5	0.9	.088
Section score	7.9	5.0	.039
Scaled section score	1.4	1.0	.111
Cognitive features			
Odd thinking/unusual perceptual			
experiences	1.4	0.8	.104
Nondelusional paranoia	1.1	0.6	.040
Quasi-psychotic thought	0.6	0.2	.055
Section score	3.1	1.6	.019
Scaled section score	1.1	0.4	.012
Impulsive features			
Substance abuse/dependency	0.6	0.2	.165
Sexual deviance	0.5	0.4	.818
Self-mutilation	1.1	0.4	.010
Manipulative suicide efforts	1.2	0.8	.272
Other (miscellaneous)			
impulsive patterns	1.3	0.9	.082
Section score	4.8	2.6	.011
Scaled section score	1.9	0.5	.001[b]
Interpersonal features			
Intolerance of aloneness	1.4	0.7	.057
Abandonment/engulfment/			
annihilation concerns	1.3	1.0	.218
Counterdependent/serious			
help/care conflict	1.6	0.9	.045
Stormy relationships	0.9	0.9	.844
Dependency/masochism	0.9	0.8	.612
Devaluation/manipulation/sadism	0.6	0.6	1.000
Demandingness/entitlement	1.2	1.0	.426
Treatment regressions	0.6	0.6	1.000
Countertransference problems	0.9	0.8	.793
Section score	9.4	7.2	.117
Scaled section score	2.4	1.6	.146
Total section scores	24.9	16.3	.010
Total scaled section scores	6.9	3.6	.002

[a] From Student's *t* test. [b] Statistically significant using Bonferroni's correction for multiple comparisons.

Table 10–4. Mean scores on Linehan's Suicidal Behaviors Questionnaire

Item description	CSA	Non-CSA	P values[a]
How often have you thought about killing yourself?	2.0	1.5	.355
How often have you thought about hurting yourself?	1.6	0.6	.031
How many times have you intentionally harmed yourself?	1.6	0.2	.061
Chances of hurting yourself in the future?	2.9	1.5	.057
Chances of hurting yourself within the next 6 months?	2.8	1.3	.043
Chances of killing yourself in the future?	2.8	2.3	.593
Chances of killing yourself in 6 months?	2.3	1.8	.498
Currently have a plan to kill/hurt yourself?	1.9	1.5	.208

[a] From Student's *t* test.

into the following five major categories: mania (manic and hypomanic episodes), all depression (major depressive, minor depressive, cyclothymia, and intermittent depressive episodes), all anxiety (panic, generalized anxiety, obsessive-compulsive, and phobic disorders), substance disorder (alcohol and drug abuse disorders), and all other psychiatric disorders (labile personality disorder, Briquet's, unspecified psychiatric disorder, and other psychiatric disorder). (There were no episodes of psychotic illnesses in either group.)

In addition, all episodes of psychiatric disorder were collapsed and compared. The two groups differed only in the RDC category Other Psychiatric Disorder. Three of the nonabused subjects met criteria under this category for bulimia, and two of the abused subjects met criteria for multiple personality disorder (MPD) ($t = 2.94$, df = 12, $P = .012$).

Further, the abused group was less likely to be rated Currently Not Mentally Ill ($t = 2.48$, df = 12, $P = .028$), meaning that more of these subjects were experiencing a current episode of psychiatric illness at the time of follow-up.

The 12 non-BPD diagnoses listed in DSM-III-R as measured by the SIDP-R were compared individually and by cluster type.

All categories were then collapsed. There were no significant differences.

There were also no significant differences in change over time between the two groups in total number of psychiatric hospitalizations or total amount of time spent in psychiatric hospitals as measured by the SADS.

Psychopathology, the McGlashan outcome measure defined as the "percentage of time subject has experienced anxiety, depression, or symptoms of emotional tension," distinguished the two groups: the abused borderline subjects showed less improvement over time ($F = 16.23$, df = 1, $P = .002$).

Social and Occupational Functioning

McGlashan's outcome measures of social activity, percentage of time employed, and global functioning over the entire follow-up interval did not differentiate the two groups.

Inspection of the means on employment showed that the nonabused group appeared to have improved more across time and that the abused group had done slightly worse (mean score CSA time 2 = 1.7 [SD = 1.2], vs. time 3 = 1.4 [SD = 1.4]; mean score non-CSA time 2 = 1.9 [SD = 1.4], vs. time 3 = 2.9 [SD = 1.2]).

In global functioning, the gains made by the nonabused group appear to be greater than those made by the abused group (mean score CSA time 2 = 1.1 [SD = 1.1], vs. time 3 = 2.3 [SD = 0.9]; non-CSA time 2 = 1.4 [SD = 0.9], vs. time 3, 3.2 [SD = 1.0]).

Of 10 potential categories rated by the SAS-SR and measuring current functioning, only the economic score indicated that the abused group was doing more poorly at time 3.

DISCUSSION

In this 7-year follow-up study of formerly hospitalized borderline patients, two subsamples of subjects, grouped according to whether they reported a history of CSA, were matched on a large number of variables.

At time 1, the abused group was disadvantaged by a history of school failure in childhood and sought psychiatric attention approximately 6 years earlier than the nonabused group. They also rated higher at time 1 on DIB items measuring substance abuse, impulsivity, experiences of depersonalization and derealization, more difficulty in interpersonal relationships, and higher overall DIB score. These findings suggest that the abused group was more impaired than the nonabused group at index admission to the study.

A parallel improvement over time was found between the abused and nonabused groups on measures of borderline diagnosis and symptomatology, other parameters of psychiatric illness, and general functioning. Similar improvements over time have been observed in long-term follow-up studies of BPD (McGlashan 1986; Paris et al. 1987; Plakun et al. 1985; Stone 1991).

On variables measuring the long-term effects of CSA over time, a difference in rate of improvement between the two groups was found on relatively few variables measuring borderline diagnosis and symptomatology. This finding was less apparent in the other two categories of outcome.

Specifically, the abused borderline subjects were more likely to retain a diagnosis of BPD based on DSM-III-R criteria (but not based on the DIB) and to rate positively for the borderline symptoms of affective instability, depression, and dysphoria or anhedonia (all at $P < .01$); and, at smaller P values, intolerance of being alone, tendencies to split staff or evoke negative countertransference reactions, and number of suicide attempts or gestures ($P < .05$).

On other parameters of psychiatric illness, the two groups were differentiated on only two items: McGlashan's outcome measure of global psychopathology and, less robustly, a negative rating for the RDC category Currently Not Mentally Ill. The RDC category Other Psychiatric Illness also distinguished the two groups: two of the abused borderline subjects met the criteria for a clinical diagnosis of MPD, and three of the nonabused borderline subjects met the criteria for a clinical diagnosis for bulimia. Although these findings cannot be taken as very robust because of the small samples and relatively small P values, the former finding is similar to those in other reports of a history of abuse (usually severe) in childhood antedating MPD (Herman et al. 1989; Stone 1991). The latter finding of more cases of bulimia in the nonabused group is in contrast to Lobel's (1992) report from cross-sectional data in which female inpatients with a history of sexual abuse were more likely to have a diagnosis of bulimia. The two groups were not differentiated on any other Axis I diagnoses, as measured by RDC, including depressive or substance abuse disorders. They were also not differentiated on any Axis II diagnoses. On variables examining social and occupational functioning, the abused borderline subjects were doing more poorly only on current economic status as scored by the SAS-SR.

Cross-sectional data at time 3 differentiated the abused from the nonabused borderline group on two instruments, again with relatively small *P* values. The abused borderline subjects scored higher on DIB-R summary statements measuring feelings of helplessness and symptoms of anxiety; transient, nondelusional paranoid experiences; a pattern of physical self-mutilation, and counterdependence in relationships. They also scored higher on the section scores of the Affect section, on both the section and scaled section scores of the Cognition and Impulse Action Patterns sections, and on the overall DIB-R scores (both unscaled and scaled). In addition, the abused borderline subjects scored higher on thoughts and chances of self-harm, but not on items measuring suicidality as measured by the SBQ.

An interesting observation was made on examining the mean values of several items from the DIB at different times. The scores for the abused group at time 3 were similar or equal to those of the nonabused group at time 1 for the following items: unstable work history, patterns of self-mutilation and substance abuse, other impulsive behaviors, Impulse Action Patterns section score, depressed or angry affect, presenting as demanding or entitled, experiences of depersonalization, Interpersonal Relationships section score, and overall DIB section score.

This pattern suggests that the abused group may be about 7 years "behind" the nonabused group in terms of certain measures of borderline psychopathology, a factor that may explain some of the differences in improvement over time between the two groups.

What seems apparent is that recovery for a borderline patient who reports a history of CSA will require more time. These patients tend to retain a DSM-III-R diagnosis of BPD, along with the specific features of dysphoria, affective instability, an intolerance for being alone, tendencies toward self-harm, and a tendency to split staff and/or evoke negative countertransference problems.

LIMITATIONS

A statistical limitation to the current study is the small sample size, suggesting low power. In addition, a history of CSA by noncaretakers was not systematically assessed, suggesting that these results represent conservative findings. The parameters of sexual abuse and other forms of childhood maltreatment or neglect, such as physical and/or psychological abuse and negative family environment, were also not systematically assessed at time 1. This limits our ability to analyze the unique, additive, and/or interactive contributions that such factors may make to the findings. Paris et al. (1993) recommended a multivariate design study in which all psychological risk factors are examined in relation to the diagnosis of BPD.

Another needed task is the measurement of mediators in childhood that have been recognized in other studies as positively affecting outcome (e.g., actual or perceived social support, maternal warmth, maternal response to the disclosure of abuse, good level of functioning in the victim's family).

Another limitation is that the sample consists of former inpatients who are predominantly female and who met criteria for BPD based on the DIB. These findings may therefore not be generalizable to less severely impaired borderline individuals or male borderline individuals.

IMPLICATIONS

These findings support the need for routine assessment of CSA in all outcome studies investigating BPD.

Future work in the current study includes the need to reassess the presence of CSA and other forms of abuse by way of a valid, reliable instrument. We are also interested in completing detailed treatment histories on subjects in order to understand whether a focus on the abuse and/or its aftereffects affects outcome. On the basis of this study, clinicians working with abused borderline patients may want to target certain aspects of psychopathology, such as tendencies toward self-harm, depressive affects, intolerance of being alone, and countertransference issues.

SUMMARY

In this follow-up study of formerly hospitalized DIB borderline patients, a history of CSA differentiated long-term outcome on a relatively small number of variables. Although the abused group was worse off to begin with, their improvement over time paralleled that of the nonabused group at 7-year follow-up. The good news for patients and clinicians alike is that, if this slope of recovery continues, there is good reason to hope that the recovery of borderline patients described in long-term follow-up studies may also apply to borderline patients who suffered sexual abuse in childhood. Our data suggest that recovery may take 5 to 10 years longer for a sexually abused borderline patient. Over the past decade, recognition of and attention to therapeutic issues related to a childhood abuse history have evolved, and we hope that this recognition and attention will augment this optimistic outlook.

REFERENCES

American Psychiatric Association: Diagnostic and Statistical Manual of Mental Disorders, 3rd Edition, Revised. Washington, DC, American Psychiatric Association, 1987

Beitchman JH, Zucker KJ, Hood JE, et al: A review of the long-term effects of child sexual abuse. Child Abuse Negl 16:101–118, 1992

Briere JN: Child Abuse Trauma: Theory and Treatment of the Lasting Effects. London, England, Sage Publications, 1992

Browne A, Finkelhor D: Impact of child sexual abuse: a review of the research. Psychol Bull 99:66–77, 1986

Dunn LM, Dunn LM: Peabody Picture Vocabulary Test—Revised. Circle Pines, MN, American Guidance Service, 1981

Endicott J, Spitzer RL: A diagnostic interview: The Schedule for Affective Disorders and Schizophrenia. Arch Gen Psychiatry 35:837–844, 1978

Gunderson JG, Kolb JE, Austin V: The Diagnostic Interview for Borderline Patients. Am J Psychiatry 138:896–903, 1981

Herman JL: Trauma and Recovery. New York, Basic Books, 1992

Herman JL, Perry JC, van der Kolk BA: Childhood trauma in borderline personality disorder. Am J Psychiatry 146:490–495, 1989

Linehan MM: Suicide Behaviors Questionnaire. Seattle, WA, University of Washington, 1983

Links PS, van Reekum R: Childhood sexual abuse, parental impairment and the development of borderline personality disorder. Can J Psychiatry 38:472–474, 1993

Links PS, Steiner M, Offord DR: Characteristics of borderline personality disorder: a Canadian study. Can J Psychiatry 33:336–340, 1988

Links PS, Mitton MJE, Steiner M: Predicting outcome for borderline personality disorder. Compr Psychiatry 31:490–498, 1990a

Links PS, Boiago I, Huxley G, et al: Sexual abuse and biparental failure as etiologic models in borderline personality disorder, in Family Environment and Borderline Personality Disorder. Edited by Links PS. Washington, DC, American Psychiatric Press, 1990b, pp 107–120

Lobel CM: Relationship between CSA and borderline personality disorder in women psychiatric inpatients. Journal of Child Sexual Abuse 1:63–80, 1992

McGlashan TH: The Chestnut Lodge follow-up study, I: follow-up methodology and study sample. Arch Gen Psychiatry 41:573–585, 1984

McGlashan TH: The Chestnut Lodge follow-up study, III: long-term outcome of borderline personality disorder. Arch Gen Psychiatry 43:20–30, 1986

Mellsop G, Peace K, Fernando T: Pre-admission adaptive functioning as a measure of prognosis in psychiatric inpatients. Aust N Z J Psychiatry 21:539–544, 1987

Paris J, Brown R, Nowlis D: Long-term follow-up of borderline patients in a general hospital. Compr Psychiatry 28:530–535, 1987

Paris J, Zweig-Frank H, Guzder H: The role of psychological risk factors in recovery from borderline personality disorder. Compr Psychiatry 34:410–413, 1993

Pfohl B, Blum N, Zimmerman M, et al: Structured Interview for DSM-III-R Personality (SIDP-R). Iowa City, IA, University of Iowa College of Medicine, Department of Psychiatry, 1989

Plakun EM, Burkhardt PE, Muller JP: 14-year follow-up of borderline and schizotypal personality disorders. Compr Psychiatry 26:448–455, 1985

Reitsma-Street M, Offord DR, Finch T: Pairs of same-sexed siblings discordant for antisocial behaviour. Br J Psychiatry 146:415–423, 1985

Schetky DH: A review of the literature on the long-term effects of CSA, in Incest-Related Syndromes of Adult Psychopathology. Edited by Kluft RP. Washington, DC, American Psychiatric Press, 1990, pp 35–54

Sheldrick C: Adult sequelae of child sexual abuse. Br J Psychiatry 138:55–62, 1991

Spitzer RL, Endicott J: Schedule for Affective Disorders and Schizophrenia, Lifetime Interval Version (SADS-LI). New York, New York State Psychiatric Institute, 1984

Spitzer RL, Endicott J, Robins E: Research Diagnostic Criteria: rationale and reliability. Arch Gen Psychiatry 35:773–782, 1978

Spitzer RL, Endicott J, Robins E: Research Diagnostic Criteria (RDC) for a Select Group of Functional Disorders, 3rd Edition, Updated. New York, New York State Psychiatric Institute, 1989

Starr RH, MacLean DJ, Keating DP: Life-span outcomes of child maltreatment, in The Effects of Child Abuse and Neglect. Edited by Starr RH, Wolfe DA. New York, Guilford, 1991, pp 1–32

Stone MH: The Fate of Borderline Patients. New York, Guilford, 1991

Weissman MM, Bothwell S: Assessment of Social Adjustment by Patient Self-Report. Arch Gen Psychiatry 33:1111–1115, 1976

Weissman M, Prusoff B, Thompson M: Social adjustment by self-report in a community sample and in psychiatric outpatients. J Nerv Ment Dis 166:317–326, 1978

Zanarini MC, Gunderson JG, Frankenburg FR, et al: The Revised Diagnostic Interview for Borderlines: discriminating BPD from other axis II disorders. Journal of Personality Disorders 3:10–18, 1989

Chapter 11

Biosocial Perspective on the Relationship of Childhood Sexual Abuse, Suicidal Behavior, and Borderline Personality Disorder

Amy W. Wagner, Ph.D., and Marsha M. Linehan, Ph.D.

I n this chapter we describe and amplify the biosocial etiological theory of borderline personality disorder (BPD) (Linehan 1987, 1993a) and the potential role of childhood sexual abuse in the development of BPD. Particular attention is given to the relationship between sexual abuse and suicidal behavior within this population. We conclude with an overview of dialectical behavior therapy for BPD, which is based on the biosocial theory, and we discuss the treatment of trauma symptoms specifically within this approach.

As discussed throughout this volume, a strong association has been demonstrated between reports of childhood sexual abuse and the diagnosis of BPD. High rates of childhood sexual abuse are reported by inpatients with the BPD diagnosis (Bryer et al. 1987; Ogata et al. 1990; Shearer et al. 1990), BPD outpatients (Herman et al. 1989; Zanarini et al. 1989), emergency room BPD patients (Briere and Zaidi 1989), and adolescent BPD populations (Goldman et al. 1992; Ludolph et al. 1990; Westen et al.

Supported in part by National Institute of Mental Health grant MH34486 to Dr. Linehan.

1990). Furthermore, degree of "borderline pathology" has been positively correlated with degree of reported childhood trauma (Herman et al. 1989) and with reports of more severe sexual abuse in general (Landecker 1992). Direct causal connections between sexual abuse and BPD are inaccurate, however, in that not all people with BPD report histories of sexual abuse, and many people who report histories of sexual abuse do not develop BPD. Questions concerning the validity of reporting obscure this relationship as well.

Rather than asserting that sexual abuse causes BPD, our group has suggested that the typical experience of childhood sexual abuse and the environment in which sexual abuse typically occurs represent the prototypic experience and environment of the individual who develops BPD. That is, the factors that typically coexist with childhood sexual abuse (environmental, interpersonal, and traumatic) are characteristic of the childhood of men and women who also develop BPD. Through a discussion of the biosocial theory of BPD, we demonstrate how these factors, plus certain predispositions, can account for the development of BPD. Thus childhood sexual abuse can be viewed as a model by which to understand the etiology of BPD, rather than as the cause per se.

BIOSOCIAL THEORY

The basic idea in the biosocial theory of BPD is that BPD arises from a combination of biologically based difficulties in the processing of emotions (i.e., in the perception of, reaction to, and modulation of emotions) plus specific environmental circumstances, as well as their transaction over time. The biological components are probably due to a combination of genetic, intrauterine, and developmental factors affecting physiological development. The environmental contributors are any circumstances that neglect, traumatize, or severely punish this emotional vulnerability specifically, or one's emotional self generally—contributors termed by Linehan the *invalidating environment* (see below).

The result of the combined biological vulnerability to emotions and the invalidating environment is a fundamental disruption of the emotion regulation system. According to the theory, emotion dysregulation in individuals with BPD consists of two factors: emotional vulnerability and deficits in the ability to regulate emotions. The components of emotional vulnerability are hypothesized to be high sensitivity to emotional stimuli, emotional intensity, and slow return to emotional baseline. High sensitivity refers to the tendency to pick up emotional cues easily, react quickly, and have a low threshold for emotional reaction. In other words, in individuals with this trait it does not take much to provoke an emotional reaction. Emotional intensity refers to extreme reactions to emotional stimuli, which frequently disrupt both cognitive processing and the ability to self-soothe. Slow return to baseline refers to reactions' being long-lasting. This trait in turn leads to narrowing of the attention toward mood-congruent aspects of the environment, biased memory, and biased interpretations (Bower 1981; Gilligan and Bower 1984), all of which contribute to maintaining the original mood state and a heightened state of arousal. Linehan views emotion dysregulation as the core pathology of BPD and views all problematic behaviors of individuals with BPD as functionally related to regulating emotions or as natural outcomes of dysregulated emotions.

The biological and environmental components of the biosocial theory are discussed next, with particular focus on the possible role of childhood sexual abuse in the development of emotion dysregulation and BPD.

Biological Factors

The biological factors influencing the development of BPD are probably varied, including genetic influences, harmful intrauterine events, and childhood environmental effects on development of the brain and nervous system. The limbic system has been most commonly associated with emotion regulation, and there are some data suggesting that borderline individuals have a low threshold for activation of limbic structures (Cowdry et al. 1985), demonstrated as high rates of complex partial seizures, episodic dyscontrol, and attention deficit disorders in this population. In addition, individuals with BPD have also been reported to have significantly more electroencephalographic (EEG) dysrhythmias than do depressed control patients (Cowdry et al. 1985; Snyder and Pitts 1984). Other studies, however, have not found differences between individuals with BPD and those with other personality disorders in prevalence of dysrhythmias, suggesting that EEG dysrhythmias may not be specific to BPD (e.g., Cornelius et al. 1989).

Two studies investigating neuropsychological testing among outpatients with BPD suggest that individuals with BPD may have neurological deficits, perhaps related to the frontal lobe. O'Leary and colleagues (1991) found that individuals with BPD had deficits in memory for complex material and for distinguishing essential from extraneous information, compared with a control group of volunteers without BPD. Similarly, Hoffman-Judd (1993) reported that outpatients with BPD had deficits in recall of complex information as well as in visuospatial tasks measuring discrimination, speed, and fluency. It is important to note, however, that some research has failed to find neurological differences between individuals with BPD and other patient populations (Cornelius et al. 1989; Ogiso 1993; Zanarini et al. 1994). More studies are clearly needed in this area.

Support for familial contributions to BPD has been suggested by several studies. It was found that the first-degree relatives of borderline patients had heightened rates of affective disorders, alcoholism and drug abuse, BPD, and closely related personality traits (see Zanarini 1993 for a review of this topic). It should be noted, however, that these positive findings do not rule out the possibility of environmental effects.

Possibilities for intrauterine effects on emotional development include malnutrition, drug and alcohol abuse, and environmental stress. The children of mothers who had these experiences demonstrated difficulties with emotion regulation similar to those of borderline individuals. For example, characteristics of fetal alcohol syndrome (resulting from excessive alcohol consumption by the mother) included hyperactivity, impulsiveness, distractibility, irritability, and sleep difficulties (Abel 1981, 1982). One study demonstrated a relationship between such intrauterine factors and BPD (see Kimble et al., Chapter 9, this volume).

Most relevant to the role of sexual abuse in a biosocial etiology of BPD are studies examining the effects of postnatal experiences on biological development. It has been well established that extreme environmental events and conditions can modify neural structures (Dennenberg 1981; Greenough 1977; Greenough et al. 1987). Recently, researchers have begun to examine the effects of childhood trauma, and of sexual abuse, specifically, on neurological development.

Hartman and Burgess (1993) proposed a thought-provoking information-processing model of the effects of sexual abuse, which asserted that the limbic system has a key role in the perception of trauma and in the short- and long-term effects of trauma. Briefly, these authors asserted that the limbic system is the primary neurological system for the integration of incoming information. When the limbic system becomes intensely activated or overwhelmed, which can be assumed to happen in many cases of sexual abuse, numbing or dissociation occurs. Chronically, this can lead to alterations in the limbic system that interact with the prefrontal cortex (Levine 1986) and can produce kindling, or sensitization to respond intensely to stimuli. In turn, according to the model, this can produce emotion dysregulation disrupting the development of neocortical pathways that affect meaning systems and the integration of experiences. In other words, sexual abuse can lead to patterns of heightened emotional arousal and emotion dysregulation in response to events or situations, which then affect subsequent perceptions, interpretations, and reactions to events or situations. This model can account for dissociative experiences, startle responses, avoidance, disrupted memory, difficulties with sexual relations, and other typical posttraumatic stress behaviors. In a sense, then, childhood trauma, and sexual abuse specifically, may actually create biological emotional vulnerability by permanently altering the central nervous system of abused children.

Two recent studies have provided preliminary support for this model. Teicher et al. (1993) investigated the relationship between childhood physical abuse and sexual abuse on limbic system functioning in adulthood, using the Limbic System Checklist-33 (LSC-33). This instrument is a self-report scale designed to measure the somatic, sensory, behavioral, and memory symptoms that occur in temporal lobe epilepsy (and thus involve the limbic system). In their sample of 253 outpatients, those who reported a history of physical abuse had a 38% increase in LSC-33 scores, those who reported sexual abuse had a 49% increase, and those who reported both types of abuse had a 113% increase. In a separate study of 115 child and adolescent psychiatric inpatients, Ito and colleagues (1993) found significantly higher rates of electrophysiological abnormalities among patients who reported abuse (psychological, physical, and sexual) compared with those who did not report abuse. Taken together, these data suggest that childhood abuse may be related to biological abnormalities, specifically within the area of the limbic system.

This biological model is quite compatible with Linehan's components of emotion dysregulation described earlier (heightened sensitivity to stimuli, intense reactions to stimuli, and slow return to baseline). Of note here is that borderline individuals reported more severe abuse, including abuse involving violence or threat, abuse that occurred over long periods, abuse by fathers or stepfathers, and abuse by more than one perpetrator, compared with other clinical and nonclinical populations (Ogata et al. 1990). Multiple types of maltreatment have also been reported at higher rates by borderline women, including physical abuse, verbal abuse, loss, and neglect (Ogata et al. 1990; Westen et al. 1990; Zanarini et al. 1989). According to the model of Hartman and Burgess (1993), these typical experiences of borderline individuals would increase the chances that kindling of the type described would occur and that central nervous system changes would result.

Invalidating Environment

Not all children who have been sexually abused or who are born with emotional sensitivity or vulnerability develop BPD. The biosocial theory of BPD asserts that this biological predisposition to emotional vulnerability becomes problematic in an environment that does not take the vulnerability into account. This is the invalidating environment. An invalidating environment, in its most essential aspect, is one that consistently communicates to the individual that his or her actions and reactions, both cognitive and emotional, are not appropriate or valid responses to events (Linehan 1993a). It is one in which the child's communication of private experiences (i.e., thoughts and feelings) are responded to with erratic, inappropriate, and extreme responses from caregivers. The expression of private experiences, particularly emotional reactions, is not validated. Instead, it is disregarded, trivialized, or punished.

A brief discussion of the facilitative effects of validating environments on emotional understanding and regulation will help highlight the harmful effects of the invalidating environment. In optimal environments, there is public validation for private experiences. This is how children learn to label, discriminate, and control emotions (Kohlenberg and Tsai 1991). For example, a child learns the concept of *sad* when the child cries and the caregiver responds "Oh, you must be sad." The caregiver may then do something soothing for the child, like rubbing his or her back. The meaning of the word *sad* and the child's ability to learn self-soothing skills both depend on the caregiver's consistently and accurately labeling and soothing the private bodily feeling of sadness (Kohlenberg and Tsai 1991). In addition, the child's private experience may inadvertently be shaped by the caregiver's reactions. For example, if a caregiver responds to crying with anger, the child may begin to experience anger or shame in response to his or her own crying. In other words, the child's actual experience of sadness may be partially altered, depending on these social reactions or contingencies.

Returning to the topic of BPD and the invalidating environment, the biosocial theory asserts that the invalidating environment disrupts the normal learning of emotional meaning, discrimination, and modulation. This environment tells the child that he or she is wrong in both the description and the analyses of his or her own experiences, and it attributes these experiences to prior personality traits rather than to the events actually precipitating them. Children in these environments may be told that they feel what they do not (e.g., "No matter what you say, you are angry"), like or prefer something they do not, or have done things they have not done. Expressions of negative emotions may be attributed to negative traits in the child—such as overreactivity, paranoia, motivation to manipulate, or lack of discipline—rather than to the event to which the child is actually reacting. Positive emotions may be viewed as silly, indiscriminate, or due to the child's age, rather than to the event. Similarly, emotional responses can be pathologized by the caregiver (e.g., "You're crazy for acting like that"). Emotionally invalidating environments are also intolerant of negative displays of emotion and place high value on pulling oneself up by the bootstraps or grinning in the face of adversity. Failure to live up to these expectations is met with criticism and disapproval.

The specific consequences of the invalidating environment, therefore, at least as hypothesized by Linehan (1993a), are the following: When the child's emotional expression fails to be validated, the child does not learn how to label private experiences and may actually come to experience emotions differently. When emotions are not acknowledged, the environment does not teach the child how to regulate them or to solve problems; furthermore, extreme emotional displays become necessary in order to evoke helpful environmental responses. When those around the child do not tolerate negative emotions and and when they oversimplify the ability to solve problems, the child does not learn how to tolerate emotions or form realistic expectations. Finally, the invalidating environment does not teach the child to trust his or her own reactions as valid, and the child, therefore, distrusts or invalidates personal experiences and relies on the environment to provide information on how to feel, think, and act.

The invalidating environment can take several forms. In the next section, we describe how childhood sexual abuse and the environment in which sexual abuse frequently occurs represent the prototypical, most extreme example of emotional invalidation and the invalidating environment. It is important to reiterate, however, that the biosocial theory does not assert that the effects of invalidation are the sole cause of BPD; BPD arises from a combination and interaction of biological and environmental circumstances, and trauma is probably one of the primary influences on the biology of individuals with BPD (although not the only possible influence).

Sexual Abuse as a Prototypical Example of Invalidation

Many theorists and researchers have written about the dynamics and family environments that accompany childhood sexual abuse, including Briere (1989, 1992), Curtois (1988), Finkelhor and Browne (1986), and Sgroi et al. (1982). We have incorporated their observations, as well as our own, into this theoretical analysis.

There are several ways in which the experience of sexual abuse can be invalidating.

First, a severe form of invalidation occurs when a child's body is "invaded," particularly when this is against the child's will and happens despite the child's efforts to avoid the abuse (Finkelhor and Browne 1986). At the level of physical sensations, it is communicated that the child's pain and discomfort are irrelevant and that the child is powerless to stop them. Not only are the child's pain and protests discounted, but it is also communicated that another person's wishes and desires are more important, and what feels to the child like his or her body to control is in fact not that at all. According to Briere (1992), this can lead to "dysfunctions of the self," where the child becomes unable to define himself or herself separately from the needs of others. From our perspective, this self-invalidation may be one of the most harmful aspects of sexual abuse, and it may be closely tied to the development of BPD, which has been conceptualized as a disorder of the self (e.g., Kernberg 1975; Masterson 1976; Wastell 1992).

Second, children are frequently given confusing messages about the meaning of the abuse (Finkelhor and Browne 1986). For example, the child may be given special attention or privileges for sexual behavior while at the same time the family and community convey that this type of behavior is wrong. Similarly, children may be told that they feel different about the abuse from they way they actually do. Examples are "you like this," when in fact it is painful or unpleasant; "you want this," when in fact the child does not; "this is OK," when society says it is not. Conversely, the sexual abuse may be experienced as pleasant or arousing, yet society says that this is not appropriate. As noted above, public validation of private experiences is needed for the child to accurately label, discriminate, and modulate emotions. Such discrepancies between private experience and public labeling make it exceedingly difficult to make sense of and regulate one's emotional experience.

Third, the abuse is often perpetrated by a person the child is dependent on or trusts, in an environment the child views as safe. Even if the abuse was not perpetrated by a trusted person, the child may feel betrayed by lack of protection from others the child does trust (e.g., family members). The experience of harm by a trusted or needed person thus invalidates the child's perception of the person and of the child's own safety (Finkelhor and Browne 1986).

Fourth, the child is usually asked or forced to keep the abuse secret (Curtois 1988). Again, the child is not provided with external validation to match internal, private experience, and the ability to understand his or her own reactions and emotions is compromised. As Curtois noted, if others do not know of the occurrence of abuse, "the child is even less prepared and must rely on the perpetrator for whatever meaning is to be given to the experience" (p. 33).

Fifth, when the abuse is disclosed, it is very common for significant others to minimize or rationalize the abuse, especially when the abuse was perpetrated by a family member (Curtois 1988). Furthermore, the child is frequently blamed for the occurrence of the abuse or for not disclosing the abuse sooner (Finkelhor and Browne 1986). Again, public reactions contradict private experiences.

In addition to the invalidating aspects of the sexually abusive experiences specifically, other characteristics of families in which sexual abuse occurs represent prototypical examples of the invalidating environment. According to Calof (1987), sexually abusive families demonstrate the following examples of invalidation: 1) lack of tolerance for differences from the family norm, especially regarding anger and conflict, 2) strong messages about the inappropriateness of sexual relations other than with a spouse, 3) neglect and lack of physical attention, except for that which occurs in the context of sexual abuse, 4) unpredictability and intermittent reinforcement, in which the child may be cared for one day and abused the next (similarly, these families are frequently chaotic—members go in and out, and substance abuse and financial problems are common), 5) violence of other types, physical abuse, and threats of abuse.

Furthermore, invalidating families appear to have more rigid and conventional rules and standards than validating families. Curtois (1988, p. 45) lists the following commonly observed standards for social interaction held by sexually abusive families:

1. Don't feel. Keep your feelings in check. Do not show your feelings, especially anger.

2. Be in control at all times. Do not show weakness. Do not ask for help.

3. Deny what is really happening. Disbelieve your own senses/perceptions. Lie to yourself and to others.

4. Don't trust yourself or anyone else. No one is trustworthy.

5. Keep the secret. If you tell, you will not be believed and you will not get help.

6. Be ashamed of yourself. You are to blame for everything.

These standards and characteristics are not only essentially invalidating of the child's experiences and wishes but are also strikingly similar to the standards reported by the BPD patients in our clinic and treatment studies—individuals both with and without histories of sexual abuse. To reiterate, the invalidating environment as described by Linehan's biosocial theory can take many forms; that is, it is not necessary to experience sexual abuse to develop BPD. Nonetheless, the characteristics of the invalidating environment overlap considerably with the common characteristics and traits evident in the environments where sexual abuse occurs and in the experience of sexual abuse itself.

The biosocial theory is a *transactional* theory. That is, the child and the environment are hypothesized to influence each other. We have been describing many of the ways in which the environment may influence the child, but there are also several ways in which the child may influence the environment. The biological predisposition to emotional vulnerability may manifest itself in ways that put the child at risk for abuse. Compared to other children, the emotionally vulnerable child may initially cry more, may have more tantrums, may seek affection more, and in general may engage in behaviors that make him or her a more salient and likely target for abuse. As the invalidating environment teaches the child that his or her thoughts, feelings, and emotions are irrelevant, the child may become less likely to complain or to disclose the abuse. In turn, the child is at higher risk of continued abuse than are other children. Unfortunately, much of what is described here is based on clinical observations only. Rigorous empirical validation of these theories is clearly needed.

DEVELOPMENT AND FUNCTION OF SUICIDAL BEHAVIOR

Suicidal behavior— including parasuicidal acts, suicide ideation, and suicide threats—is very common in individuals diagnosed with BPD, and it has been shown to discriminate BPD from all other personality disorders (Gunderson 1984; Morey 1988; Zanarini et al. 1990). Interestingly, recent studies also link suicidal behavior to histories of childhood sexual abuse. Among outpatients who report histories of sexual abuse, rates of previous parasuicide range from 33% to 55%, compared to 5%–34% for those who do not report abuse (Bagley and Ramsay 1985; Briere 1984, 1988; Briere and Runtz 1986; Herman and Hirschman 1981; Sedney and Brooks 1984). Indeed, Landecker (1992) suggested that suicidal behavior in individuals with BPD may be related to the traumatic aspects of childhood experiences and to sexual abuse specifically. The biosocial theory predicts that this relationship would evolve in the following ways.

Suicidal Behavior as an Emotion Regulator

Suicidal behavior is perhaps one of the most effective ways in which borderline individuals have learned to regulate painful or overwhelming negative emotions. Many individuals have reported in retrospect that the intent of the parasuicidal behavior, including suicide attempts, was to escape or end their painful feelings, including shame, anxiety, and anger. For example, in response to overdosing, many individuals sleep or experience deep physiological relaxation. This may provide temporary respite from emotions, and the sleep or rest may actually reduce the intensity of the emotions. Self-mutilation—for example, cutting and burning—also have powerful emotion regulation effects. It is unclear what physiological mechanisms are affected by these acts, but many borderline individuals report substantial relief from intense emotions after engaging in these behaviors. Furthermore, many borderline individuals report that suicidal behavior helps them to stop dissociating, which often occurs in response to painful emotions.

Landecker (1992) reviewed studies showing, interestingly, that individuals who experienced sexual abuse (and do not meet criteria for BPD) and rape victims reported similar emotion regulation effects from parasuicidal behavior. Examples of specific reasons given for engaging in the behavior among these populations include a "means to relieve overwhelming and painful tension," "an attempt to end these frightening depersonalized feelings," and the result of an "inability to express feelings verbally" (all quotations from p. 237).

Suicidal Behavior as a Means of Getting Help

Both suicide threats and parasuicidal acts are also very effective in getting help from the environment, which can have the result of reducing painful emotions. In the invalidating environment, less extreme requests for help may be ineffective. To get help, the borderline individual must act in an extreme manner, and suicidal behavior gets attention. As an example, one of our patients reported that she "went crazy" (i.e., started cutting herself) in order to go to the hospital and escape the sexual abuse from her father. Over time, with few other skills by which to seek help, these extreme behaviors become reinforced. Indeed, suicidal behavior is one of the most effective ways that nonpsychotic individuals have of being admitted to the hospital. Similarly, suicidal behavior is reinforced by many therapists who tell their patients to contact them only in an emergency; feeling suicidal is commonly viewed as a qualifying emergency.

We now provide a brief overview of Linehan's cognitive-behavior therapy for borderline personality disorder, dialectical behavior therapy (DBT) (the interested reader is referred to the treatment manual and associated updates for a fuller description [Linehan 1993a, 1993b]). This therapy was designed to treat the problematic behaviors associated with emotion dysregulation in borderline individuals and has been demonstrated to effectively reduce suicidal behavior specifically in this population (Linehan et al. 1991). Because a thorough description of DBT is not possible here, we focus on the treatment of sexual abuse (and other past traumatic experiences) specifically within DBT.

DIALECTICAL BEHAVIOR THERAPY

As stated, DBT is, at its core, a cognitive-behavior therapy. As with standard behavior therapies, DBT presumes that attention to both skill acquisition and behavioral motivation is essential for change. In developing DBT, however, standard behavior therapies proved insufficient in treating borderline patients, for the following reasons:

1) Focusing on patient change, either in motivation or by enhancing skills, is often experienced as invalidating by traumatized individuals and precipitates withdrawal, noncompliance, and at times, early dropout from treatment. 2) Skills training to the extent believed necessary is extraordinarily difficult, if not impossible, within the context of a therapy oriented to reducing borderline behavioral patterns, including behaviors that are definite sequelae of traumatic experiences. 3) Similarly, sufficient attention to motivational issues cannot be given in a treatment with a set skill-training agenda. 4) New behavioral coping skills are difficult to remember and apply when one is in a state of crisis, making generalization of skills to other situations difficult. 5) Traumatized and borderline individuals often unwittingly reinforce therapists for iatrogenic treatment and punish them for effective treatment strategies.

To take these factors into account, Linehan (1993a) made three modifications to standard behavior therapy. First, a number of treatment strategies that better reflect acceptance and validation of the patient's current capacities and behavioral functioning were gathered and added to the treatment. The dialectical philosophical emphasis of the treatment ensures the balance of acceptance and change within the treatment as a whole and within each individual interaction. Second, treatment of the patient was split into three components: one that focuses primarily on skill acquisition, one that focuses primarily on motivational issues and skill strengthening, and one designed explicitly to foster generalization of skills to everyday life outside the treatment context. Third, a consultation/team meeting with specific guidelines for keeping the therapist within the treatment frame was added.

In standard outpatient DBT, treatment consists of structured psychosocial individual or group therapy (for skills training), individual psychotherapy (addressing motivational and skills strengthening), telephone contact with the individual therapist (addressing generalization), and peer supervision meetings (to treat the therapist). On a psychiatric inpatient or day treatment unit, the coaching might be done by the milieu; in community mental health settings, it might be done by after-hours teams or crisis phone workers. DBT is further characterized by the biosocial theoretical perspective described above, a philosophy of dialectics, a clear hierarchy of treatment targets (the behaviors identified for change), and a set of treatment strategy groups (tactics and procedures of the therapist used to achieve change). In contrast to many behavioral approaches, DBT also places great emphasis on the therapeutic relationship.

As with other therapeutic orientations, Linehan divides therapy into several discrete stages. The division, however, is largely for heuristic purposes, because therapeutic progress usually occurs in a recursive fashion, with constant movement to previous stages and jumps to subsequent stages. Because DBT requires a voluntary, collaborative therapeutic relationship, the first stage of treatment is considered a pretreatment stage; the focuses are orientation to treatment and commitment to goals and to therapy. During this pretreatment phase, the therapist assists the patient in making an informed decision about committing to therapy and also obtains sufficient information about the patient to decide whether the therapist can work with the patient. Generally, in DBT, the minimum patient commitment is agreement by the patient that a goal of treatment is to replace maladaptive coping styles—including suicidal behaviors and impulsive dropping out of treatment—with skillful coping behaviors. In this context, the patient and therapist must make a (usually renewable) time-limited commitment to work together. The patient agrees to come to psychotherapy (or whatever primary mode of treatment is offered) and to actively participate in learning new behavioral skills, and the therapist agrees to offer the treatment and to be available for coaching on a reasonable schedule.

Stage 1 of DBT has as its primary focus the attainment of basic living capacities. During this phase, the targets of therapy are 1) reducing suicidal behaviors, 2) building a collaborative therapeutic relationship, 3) reducing major behavior patterns that make it impossible to have a life of reasonable quality (e.g., serious substance abuse, homelessness, frequent psychiatric hospitalizations, inability to hold a job or maintain a friendship), and 4) building skills for distress tolerance, interpersonal effectiveness, emotion regulation, self-management, and the ability to control unwanted mental activities (mindfulness skills). In general, these targets are approached hierarchically: behaviors early in this list (e.g., suicidal behavior) are worked on first until they are no longer problematic.

Stage 2, entered only after there is sufficient progress in stage 1, involves direct focus on emotionally processing past traumatic events. During this stage, exposure-based strategies are used to prompt remembering, describing, analyzing, experiencing, and desensitizing to any previous traumatic events of consequence. For individuals who have been sexually and physically abused or neglected during childhood, these events will usually take up a significant portion of this phase of treatment. However, as we noted previously, the biosocial theory of BPD offered by Linehan does not presume that abuse per se is the necessary condition for development of BPD. Invalidation, especially when it represents a threat to the individual's sense of personal integrity, is the presumed etiological condition. Thus, during stage 2, the DBT therapist helps the patient emotionally process previous experiences of serious or consequential invalidation, whether or not actual abusive behavior (in the usual sense of that word) occurred. This processing includes validation of the original events and their attendant affects and validation of the sense of outrage and disappointment that these events were initially ignored.

Because of its emphasis on exposure and emotional processing, stage 2 of DBT is similar, if not identical at times, to other treatments, including the exposure-based treatment developed by behavior therapists (e.g., Foa et al. 1991), the uncovering treatments proposed by psychodynamic therapists (e.g., Herman 1992), and the trauma-specific treatments developed by Briere (1989, 1992).

Emotional processing of traumatic experiences occurs in stage 2 of DBT primarily because it is crucial that patients first learn the skills to cope with the intense emotions evoked in the course of this work (e.g., emotion regulation and distress tolerance skills). Without these skills, patients may resort to the maladaptive ways they had learned to cope in the past—for example, suicidal behavior, drugs and alcohol, and dissociation. It is important to note, however, that histories of sexual abuse, physical abuse, emotional abuse, neglect, and other forms of invalidation are always assessed early in treatment. It is further explained to patients that these experiences are important and may be discussed later in treatment, but first the focus will be on developing basic living capacities in order to make processing of these experiences possible.

This is not to imply that patients' reports of abuse or trauma are ignored in stage 1 of DBT, because it is quite common for patients to report memories or flashbacks during this time. Abuse may be discussed during stage 1 to the extent that it is relevant to the target behavior. For example, a precipitant to suicidal behavior might be flashbacks of abuse. Therapy may then focus on developing ways other than suicidal behavior to cope with these flashbacks.

Overlapping with the first two stages, and forming the final stage of therapy, is a focus on developing the ability to trust the self; to validate one's own opinions, emotions, and actions; and in general to respect oneself independently of the therapist and of other people. As discussed earlier, these issues are central for individuals who have experienced severe invalidation, and sexual abuse specifically. Stage 3, therefore, focuses on increasing self-respect and achieving individual goals of the patient. The goal here is to "be able to rely on oneself while remaining firmly within reciprocal interpersonal networks" (Linehan 1993a,

p. 173). Thus, a further goal is to strengthen the patient's sense of personal connection to the present—connections that either were never formed or were severed during traumatic episodes. Enhancing self-respect also requires the reduction of residual self-hate and shame that often remains after desensitization to abuse memories. Termination from intensive therapy (but not necessarily from the therapist or from intermittent therapy sessions) is also accomplished during this stage.

CONCLUSION

We have described Linehan's biosocial theory of the etiology of BPD, the role of sexual abuse specifically within this population, and Linehan's cognitive-behavior treatment for BPD. The major premises are that a necessary component in the development of BPD is an invalidating environment and that childhood sexual abuse represents a prototypical example of extreme invalidation. However, sexual abuse per se may or may not be present, because invalidation can take many forms. This theory has important implications for clinicians working with borderline patients. It is not uncommon for professionals to question the reliability of borderline patients' reports of abuse. In contrast, the biosocial theory asserts that if extreme or pervasive invalidation did occur, the actual form the invalidation took is, in a sense, irrelevant. The risk of disbelieving the borderline patient is that the therapist may potentially re-create the invalidating environment. Furthermore, as reported in many different contexts in this volume, there is extensive research linking reports of childhood sexual abuse and the development of BPD, and no research to date suggests that these reports are inaccurate.

REFERENCES

Abel EL: Behavioral teratology of alcohol. Psychol Bull 50:564–581, 1981

Abel EL: Consumption of alcohol during pregnancy: a review of effects on growth and development of offspring. Hum Biol 54:421–453, 1982

Bagley C, Ramsay R: Disrupted childhood and vulnerability to sexual assault: long-term sequels with implications for counseling. Journal of Social Work and Human Sexuality 4:33–48, 1985

Bower GH: Mood and memory. Am Psychol 36:129–148, 1981

Briere J: The effects of childhood sexual abuse on later psychological functioning: defining a "post-sexual-abuse syndrome." Paper presented at the Third National Conference on Sexual Victimization of Children, Washington, DC, April 1984

Briere J: The long-term clinical correlates of childhood sexual victimization. Ann N Y Acad Sci 528:327–334, 1988

Briere J: Therapy for Adults Molested as Children: Beyond Survival. New York, Springer, 1989

Briere J: Child Abuse Trauma: Theory and Treatment of the Lasting Effects. Newbury Park, CA, Sage, 1992

Briere J, Runtz M: Suicidal thoughts and behaviours in former sexual abuse victims. Canadian Journal of Behavioural Sciences 18:413–423, 1986

Briere J, Zaidi LY: Sexual abuse histories and sequelae in female psychiatric emergency room patients. Am J Psychiatry 146:1602–1606, 1989

Bryer JB, Nelson BA, Miller JB, et al: Childhood sexual and physical abuse as factors in adult psychiatric illness. Am J Psychiatry 144:1426–1430, 1987

Calof D: Treating adult survivors of incest and child abuse. Workshop presented at The Family Network Symposium, Washington, DC, 1987

Cornelius JR, Soloff PH, George AWA, et al: An evaluation of the significance of selected neuropsychiatric abnormalities in the etiology of borderline personality disorder. Journal of Personality Disorders 3:19–25, 1989

Cowdry RW, Pickar D, Davies R: Symptoms and EEG findings in the borderline syndrome. Int J Psychiatry Med 15:201–211, 1985

Curtois CA: Healing the Incest Wound: Adult Survivors in Therapy. New York, WW Norton, 1988

Dennenberg VH: Hemispheric laterality in animals and the effects of early experience. Behavioral and Brain Sciences 4:1–49, 1981

Finkelhor D, Browne A: Initial and long-term effects: a conceptual framework, in A Sourcebook on Child Sexual Abuse. Edited by Finkelhor D. Newbury Park, CA, Sage, 1986, pp 180–198

Foa EB, Rothbaum BO, Riggs D, et al: Treatment of post-traumatic stress disorder in rape victims. J Consult Clin Psychol 59:715–723, 1991

Gilligan SG, Bower GH: Cognitive consequences of emotional arousal, in Emotions, Cognition, and Behavior. Edited by Izard CE, Kagan J, Zajonc RB. Cambridge, England, Cambridge University Press, 1984, pp 547–588

Goldman SJ, D'Angelo EJ, DeMaso DR, et al: Physical and sexual abuse histories among children with borderline personality disorder. Am J Psychiatry 149:1723–1726, 1992

Greenough WT: Experimental modification of the developing brain, in Current Trends in Psychology. Edited by Janis IL. Los Altos, CA, William Kaufmann, 1977, pp 82–90

Greenough WT, Black JE, Wallace CS: Experience and brain development. Child Dev 58:539–559, 1987

Gunderson J: Borderline Personality Disorder. Washington, DC, American Psychiatric Press, 1984

Hartman CR, Burgess AW: Information processing of trauma. Child Abuse Negl 17:47–58, 1993

Herman JL: Trauma and Recovery. New York, Basic Books, 1992

Herman JL, Hirschman L: Families at risk for father-daughter incest. Am J Psychiatry 138:967–979, 1981

Herman JL, Perry JC, van der Kolk BA: Childhood trauma in borderline personality disorder. Am J Psychiatry 146:490–495, 1989

Hoffman-Judd P: Neuropsychological dysfunction in borderline personality disorder. Paper presented at the Third International Congress on the Disorders of Personality, Cambridge, MA, September 1993

Ito Y, Teicher MH, Glod CA, et al: Increased prevalence of electrophysiological abnormalities in children with psychological, physical, and sexual abuse. J Neuropsychiatry Clin Neurosci 5:401–408, 1993

Kernberg OF: Borderline Conditions and Pathological Narcissism. New York, Jason Aronson, 1975

Kohlenberg RJ, Tsai M: Functional Analytic Psychotherapy: Creating Intense and Curative Therapeutic Relationships. New York, Plenum, 1991

Landecker H: The role of childhood sexual trauma in the etiology of borderline personality disorder: considerations for diagnosis and treatment. Psychotherapy 29:234–242, 1992

Levine P: Stress, in Psychophysiology: Systems, Processes and Applications. Edited by Coles M, Donchin E, Porges S. New York, Guilford, 1986, pp 331–353

Linehan MM: Dialectical behavior therapy for borderline personality disorder. Bull Menninger Clin 51:261–276, 1987

Linehan MM: Cognitive-Behavioral Treatment for Borderline Personality Disorder. New York, Guilford, 1993a

Linehan MM: Skills Training Manual for Treatment of Borderline Personality Disorder. New York, Guilford, 1993b

Linehan MM, Armstrong HE, Suarez A, et al: Cognitive-behavioral treatment of chronically parasuicidal borderline patients. Arch Gen Psychiatry 48:1060–1064, 1991

Ludolph PS, Westen D, Misle B, et al: The borderline diagnosis in adolescents: symptoms and developmental history. Am J Psychiatry 147:470–476, 1990

Masterson JF: Psychotherapy of the Borderline Adult: A Developmental Approach. New York, Brunner/Mazel, 1976

Morey LC: A psychometric analysis of the DSM-III-R personality disorder criteria. Journal of Personality Disorders 2:109–124, 1988

Ogata SN, Silk KR, Goodrich S, et al: Childhood sexual and physical abuse in adult patients with borderline personality disorder. Am J Psychiatry 147:1008–1013, 1990

Ogiso Y: Relationship between clinical symptoms and EEG findings in borderline personality disorder. Paper presented at the Third International Congress on the Disorders of Personality, Cambridge, MA, September 1993

O'Leary KM, Brouwers P, Gardner DL: Neuropsychological testing of patients with borderline personality disorder. Am J Psychiatry 148:106–111, 1991

Sedney MA, Brooks B: Factors associated with a history of childhood sexual experience in a nonclinical female population. J Am Acad Child Adolesc Psychiatry 23:215–218, 1984

Sgroi SM, Blick LC, Porter FS: A conceptual framework for child sexual abuse, in Handbook of Clinical Intervention in Child Sexual Abuse. Edited by Sgroi SM. Lexington, MA, Lexington Books, 1982, pp 9–37

Shearer SL, Peters CP, Quaytman MS, et al: Frequency and correlates of childhood sexual and physical abuse histories in adult female borderline inpatients. Am J Psychiatry 147:214–216, 1990

Snyder S, Pitts WM: Electroencephalography of DSM-III borderline personality disorder. Acta Psychiatr Scand 69:129–134, 1984

Teicher MH, Glod CA, Surrey J, et al: Early childhood abuse and limbic system ratings in adult psychiatric outpatients. J Neuropsychiatry Clin Neurosci 5:301–306, 1993

Wastell CA: Self psychology and the etiology of borderline personality disorder. Psychotherapy 29:225–233, 1992

Westen D, Ludolph P, Misle B, et al: Physical and sexual abuse in adolescent girls with borderline personality disorder. Am J Orthopsychiatry 60:55–66, 1990

Zanarini MC: BPD as an impulse spectrum disorder, in Borderline Personality Disorder: Etiology and Treatment. Edited by Paris J. Washington, DC, American Psychiatric Press, 1993, pp 67–85

Zanarini MC, Gunderson JG, Marino MF, et al: Childhood experiences of borderline patients. Compr Psychiatry 30:18–25, 1989

Zanarini MC, Gunderson JG, Frankenburg FR, et al: Discriminating borderline personality disorder from other Axis II disorders. Am J Psychiatry 147:161–167, 1990

Zanarini MC, Kimble CR, Williams AA: Neurological dysfunction in borderline patients and Axis II control subjects, in Biological and Neurobehavioral Studies of Borderline Personality Disorder. Edited by Silk KR. Washington, DC, American Psychiatric Press, 1994, pp 159–175

Chapter 12

Effects of a History of Childhood Abuse on Treatment of Borderline Patients

John G. Gunderson, M.D.

O ur understanding of the etiology, psychopathology, and course of borderline personality disorder (BPD) and of the treatment of patients with the disorder has grown dramatically as a result of research conducted in the past 15 years. Previously, borderline psychopathology was conceptualized as a form of personality organization, and virtually all treatments involved long-term psychoanalytic therapies. However, the borderline construct has been revised to the extent that it is now recognized as a form of personality disorder, with a complicated biogenetic substrate and multifactorial environmental contributions. It is also recognized that a wide range of treatments, most of them focused and of defined length, can be beneficial (Gunderson and Links 1995).

In the course of the last decade, in which psychiatric and public attention have been drawn to the high prevalence and clinical significance of childhood sexual abuse, the borderline disorder has been singled out for having an especially high frequency of such histories. Beginning with the seminal research by Herman et al. (1989), Links et al. (1988), and Zanarini et al. (1989), a large amount of research has concentrated on the role that such abuse plays in the pathogenesis of this disorder. Such research has documented that approximately 60% of borderline patients will have a history of childhood sexual or physical abuse and that such patients have more dissociative and self-mutilative experiences than borderline patients without this history (Gunderson and Sabo 1993).

Chu and I recently described some of the treatment implications for patients with BPD of having a trauma history (Gunderson and Chu 1993). This chapter reflects many of the perspectives reported there, but here I also discuss other implications, as well as some modifications in my thinking based on still growing experience with such patients. In particular, more attention is given here to the problems associated with overreactions to abuse histories and how such histories lend themselves to using cognitive-behavioral strategies.

OVERALL STRATEGY

Treatment planning for all borderline patients should develop out of a recognition that their treatment needs are long term and are likely to involve recurrent crises. Such an overview is particularly important for borderline patients who have childhood abuse histories, both because their prognosis is generally worse and because the crises are likely to differ in some particular ways. Borderline patients who have childhood abuse histories will have more dissociative experiences, more repetitious self-mutilation, and a worse prognosis. (See Zweig-Frank and Paris, Chapter 6, and Dubo et al., Chapter 7, this volume, for a fuller discussion of the relationship of abuse to core areas of borderline symptomatology; see Mitton et al., Chapter 10, this volume, for a fuller discussion of the relationship of abuse to the course of BPD.) Moreover, the difficulties for such patients in allying themselves stably with therapeutic objectives or with therapists, as well as the importance of their accomplishing such alliances, will be magnified.

The development of an alliance for these patients is often facilitated by a clinician's managerial skill as much as his or her understanding. The patient first needs to learn that a therapist is reliable and nonpunitive. Thus, I believe the overall treatment planning for a borderline patient with an abuse history should be anchored by contacts with a single caretaker who oversees the treatment and gets involved in helping the patient manage his or her life. During this process an increasingly trusting relationship forms. This relationship can help assuage anxieties, provide direction and feedback, and can be the prototype for a more trusting relationship with an authority figure and a more secure form of attachment to a caretaker. The acquisition of the ability to have such a relationship eventually may lend itself to the patient's ability to do exploratory psychotherapy.

THE CLINICIAN-MANAGER

The abused borderline patient is particularly intolerant of interventions that are the staples of dynamic psychotherapy (i.e., interpretation and confrontation). Interpretation of the unconscious or enacted motives or meaning is often experienced as blaming or intrusive and can lead to flight or negative therapeutic reactions. Confrontation brings to attention unpleasant realities that the patient has avoided and that are often overwhelming.

The earlier era, in which the widely advocated methods of dynamic therapy were described, was usually set in a context of prolonged residential care that offered patients supports by which to process such stress. Such environments also actively encouraged patients to learn more adaptive social and vocational skills, which may even then have been more important aspects of such treatment programs than were psychotherapeutic insights. Modern borderline patients, especially those with childhood abuse, are often too buffeted by situational crises and lack of sufficient social supports to find the exploratory process meaningful. The modern therapist finds that such borderline patients usually need to be seen primarily in an outpatient context and that they need to address the immediate problems of adequate living situations, health hazards, absent vocational skills, and lack of social supports. Additionally, these issues need to be addressed without the help of a multidisciplinary treatment team. To provide meaningful help to such patients, the modern clinician will need to forgo psychodynamic interventions and adopt new and more varied forms of assistance that help patients manage their daily lives.

Among the most important undertakings for the clinician-manager will be to help the patient diminish sources of stress and improve his or her ways of coping with stressors. To do this, the clinician-manager will have to borrow tools from community-based social psychiatry and from cognitive-behavior therapists.

DEVELOPING AN ALLIANCE

Development of a reasonably stable therapeutic alliance is a critically important, but very difficult, task in the early phase of working with borderline patients. Although recent studies have shown that the level of alliance that borderline patients give to their therapist varies greatly even within a given therapeutic hour (Gabbard et al. 1988), our research has shown that for those who remain in therapy, the alliance will gradually improve over the course of years (J. G. Gunderson, L. M. Najavits, and C. N. Begin, "An empirical study of the therapeutic alliance in borderline patients," unpublished manuscript, January 1996).

The borderline patient's account of childhood abuse experiences can be of particular importance in the development of an alliance. As noted previously, validating the experience of being abused is a very important aspect of helping such patients to feel cared for and to develop a positive attachment to a therapist (Gunderson and Chu 1993). Yet this "validation" should be separated from accepting the literal truth of such accounts. In clinical work, most badly abused patients are sufficiently fractured that self-care and survival issues predominate. For more coherent patients who are quite vocal about the failures of caretakers and who seem particularly eager to talk about past mistreatment, it is wise to remain a concerned but neutral listener. The eagerness of borderline patients to report such mistreatment is sometimes greeted by an equally eager but reflexive validation that ignores the here-and-now transference significance of the reasons for their wanting to tell about such abuse.

Although it is important to suspend disbelief, it is also important not to become an unobjective listener who assumes the literal validity of those abuse accounts. The high level of public consciousness about childhood abuse and the outraged concern for its victims has been magnified within mental health services. In particular, the intense need of borderline patients for nurturant attention will fuel their reporting of abusive experiences. Moreover, the embellishment of such accounts can be aided by the borderline patient's vulnerabilities in both reality testing and reality sense.

Several well-publicized cases have highlighted the problems associated with a noncritical belief in a borderline patient's accounts of childhood abuse. Although it is easy for me, and I expect for most clinicians, to isolate these cases as reflecting only on the misjudgments of the therapists involved in them, they contain some broader truths that, in less dramatic ways, many clinicians choose to ignore. Among the truths are these: clinicians need to keep a wary eye on countertransference sources for their sympathetic responses to a patient's accounts of childhood abuse, and clinicians need to be aware of the potential hazards deriving from their perceptions of the patient as a victim and the family as cruel and sadistic. Some of the misguided consequences of ignoring such countertransference reactions are premature efforts to get patients to renounce or leave their families or spouses, exaggerated fears about abandoning patients (based on the belief in one's being irreplaceable), and the failure to invoke and use the parents as important resources.

SOCIOTHERAPIES

It is important for the clinician-manager to identify the sources of stress in the abused borderline patient's life that are responsible for his or her crises and self-mutilative acts. This will often involve assessing the patient's major relationships. Here the clinician-manager should be willing to hold, and should even encourage, conjoint meetings involving the borderline patient and significant others. If the patient is still financially or emotionally dependent on the parents, it is often helpful to meet with the parents and provide them with a psychoeducation about the nature of borderline psychopathology. Unfortunately, the attention given to abuse as a pathogenic factor in the development of BPD has discouraged clinicians from involving families. This is so because in the service of being empathic, clinicians have tacitly accepted vilification of families. Most of the time, abuse occurred long before the treatment, and in many of these instances, the parents' role was passive—failing to recognize or to prevent the abuse. It is very rare that a borderline patient's report of abuse should prevent efforts to involve and educate family members on whom the patient is dependent.

Within the context of psychosocial meetings with significant others, I believe it can be helpful to identify the deficits that borderline patients have as a way of evoking a more supportive set of responses by those with whom they live. Briefly, the identification of a deficit in impulse/affect regulation provides a framework from which significant others can make efforts to avoid the types of angry, critical, and rejecting responses that stimulate such intense affective responses and frequently the impulsive acting out of such affects. Identification of the cognitive deficit called *splitting*, or the tendency toward dichotomous thinking, can help significant others to offer more modulated and cautious reactions to reports either of having been cruelly mistreated or of having found a perfect healer. Identification of the deficit in tolerating aloneness can help others to anticipate the problems surrounding separations and the importance their borderline relative attaches to sustaining relationships and contacts with others.

Notably, these meetings with the abused borderline patient's significant others should not be construed as either couples therapy or family therapy. Not only does that construction invite resistance to participation on the part of the significant others, but it also suggests that the purpose of the meetings will be to explore others' relationships with the borderline patient. In contrast, the purpose of these meetings is to provide information to the significant others in ways that will actively help them be less stressful to the borderline patient. When meetings are offered from this perspective, borderline patients who would otherwise resist such meetings will often be grateful for this form of outreach.

Other forms of sociopsychiatric intervention derive from abused borderline patients' needs to learn how to take care of themselves. The traditional concern with diminishing self-destructiveness should be emphasized less than the importance of social rehabilitation, in the forms of groups and vocational rehabilitation programs. Whether abused or not, borderline patients frequently have failed histories of employment, and these failures are frequently due to concerns about competence and independence. Issues of competence can be addressed directly by involvement in training programs or sheltered work programs, and encouragement and direction to do so should be followed by giving the same attention to the problems encountered therein that one would give to silence or provocative behaviors.

As noted in the earlier study (Gunderson and Chu 1993), groups may play a particularly important role for borderline patients with serious abuse histories. Such groups should not be directed at interpersonal processes and the expression of feelings—which, like exploratory psychotherapy, are likely to be overwhelming. Rather, the groups appropriate for traumatized borderline patients are those focusing on coping skills and practical solutions to current problems—that is, the very orientation proposed here for the early stage of individual "psychotherapy" itself. The benefits of such group involvement will not, then, involve insights or affect regulation, but rather a sense of group connection and diminished isolation.

COGNITIVE-BEHAVIORAL INTERVENTIONS

Westen (1991) points out that much of what has been called supportive psychotherapy involves interventions akin to those traditionally employed by cognitive-behavior therapists. Thus, for example, with respect to splitting, helping the patient realize that he saw the therapist as someone quite different before a current idealization or devaluation can be done by interpretation, by educative clarification, or by identifying these as dichotomous cognitive schemas. Through any of these techniques, the patient learns to become more self-observing. Westen goes on to cite Meichenbaum's (1977) approach to teaching impulse control by directions to stop, look, listen, delay, plan, and implement a response as directions that, when concretely provided by therapists, can gradually become internalized by the patient. He proposes that borderline patients can learn to identify and name their maladaptive patterns of thinking or perceiving, even as they occur, and that upon identifying these patterns, the patients will stop and delay proceeding with their usual behavioral response until they have considered its consequences.

Clinicians who are interested in developing such skills for the early phase of therapy with borderline patients will want to read the accounts by Beck and Freeman (1990) and Young (1990). These authors have identified maladaptive cognitive schemas that they believe are specific to borderline patients and that they believe can be modified by cognitive therapy methods. For example, borderline patients can be taught that they have a problem with dichotomous (all-or-none, black-or-white) thinking, and they can be helped to become aware of how this prejudices their judgments and causes them problems. For example, a patient who is thinking that somebody is wonderful will be enjoined to stop and think of this as evidence of his inability to see gray zones—and as a warning signal that he is likely to be overlooking the inevitable flaws of that person. Similarly, when a patient finds herself mistrusting someone, she will be enjoined to consider that this is probably a product of her disturbed perceptions and that she has reason to think she may exaggerate the malevolent intentions of others too quickly.

Linehan's (1987) behavioral therapy centers on the borderline patient's primary dysregulation of emotions. Linehan advocates a directive, intervention-oriented, proactive, problem-solving orientation. Although it involves sympathetic acknowledgment of the patient's sense of desperation, such acknowledgment is followed by proactive, relatively emotionally neutral efforts to dissect problems and plan improved ways of coping, and therapy includes rehearsals, homework, and reporting back. This approach has now been shown to be effective in diminishing deliberate self-harm and hospitalizations, and (equally impressive to me) it has been shown to engage borderline patients in the therapy so effectively that the frequency of dropouts is greatly diminished (Linehan et al. 1991). The roughly 14% of patients who drop out of treatment compares favorably with the more than 50% found to drop out of usual outpatient psychotherapies (Gunderson et al. 1989; Skodol et al. 1983). Indeed, patients' remaining in the behavioral treatment in the numbers they did may account for diminished self-destructiveness as much as do the specific behavioral techniques. If this is the case, it supports the fact that clinicians can learn from these methods about how to engage and sustain their borderline patients in treatment. This is not a trivial concern, because research suggests that borderline patients who remain in therapy for longer periods are more likely to improve (L. Hoke, "Longitudinal Patterns of Behaviors in Borderline Personality Disorder," unpublished doctoral dissertation, Boston University, 1989; Howard et al. 1986).

What I believe is the more general truth shown by cognitive-behavioral strategies for borderline patients is that a proactive, focused approach to problems that sidesteps both the exploration of the relationship and the expression of feelings may help borderline patients ally with and trust their treaters. Such an approach may also diminish many of the intense countertransference responses occurring when therapists become projective targets. Patients' projections are encouraged when a therapist assumes either a more neutral or a more passive role.

From the abused borderline patients' point of view, they enjoy the experience of someone who is actively working with them to solve problems, even when the efforts fail; and in this process, the patients more quickly come to trust the good intentions of the therapist than they otherwise would.

All borderline patients, in my experience, need to test whether the commitment and readiness to assume some kind of active, protective role in their care is present. With the incorporation of cognitive-behavioral approaches, the same testing will occur, but it is likely to be repeated less often. It is also likely to be less dangerous—because the therapist is openly prepared to intervene on the patient's behalf and because the therapist makes conscious and open efforts not to be a blank screen inviting projections.

DYNAMIC PSYCHOTHERAPY

What then is the role of dynamic psychotherapy in the overall treatment of the traumatized borderline patient? First of all, it should be noted 1) that there is a considerable range of trauma in the background of borderline patients and 2) that the managerial approach discussed is going to be both more necessary and more prolonged for those who have the more serious fractures in their personality as a result of their abuse—and for the borderline patients, abused or otherwise, who have the fewest social support resources. Nonetheless, dynamic psychotherapy is a form of treatment whose particular emphasis on exploration, self-disclosure, expression of affects, and understanding of unconscious motives, especially as they emerge in the transference, will almost always need to be employed judiciously until borderline patients have stabilized their life situation and developed a positive alliance with the therapist. Ideally, the early processes of stabilization and alliance building can and should be accompanied by interpretations of the motives behind a patient's maladaptive actions. However, learning from such interpretations is a secondary goal, and the requisite dynamic understanding is often unavailable.

Both the personality and the training of the clinicians who are best at engaging and making alliances with borderline patients may be quite different from those factors in clinicians who are best at psychoanalytic therapy. Clinicians who are most able to engage and make alliances with abused borderline patients will often have had a considerable amount of experience in working with such patients and will, by their nature, be practical and active. Although psychodynamic understanding may be an asset, it is neither necessary nor even necessarily helpful. Inexperienced and nonprofessional people can learn to serve as such an anchor, but they will need to have close, ongoing supervision to retain calm reasonableness during the course of crises. To do the analytic work that may render patients effectively nonborderline requires psychodynamic sophistication and a tolerance for one's own and others' aggression.

The exploration of negative hostility in the transference has seemed central to the psychotherapeutic processes that transform the structures of the borderline personality so as to render such people essentially nonborderline. As noted elsewhere (Gunderson et al. 1993; Waldinger and Gunderson 1987), the working through of negative transference rarely occurs before the third year of continuous dynamic psychotherapy, held at least twice a week. Chu and I also noted that the working through, in terms of reexperiencing and recall of memories related to childhood abuse, is a part of individual psychotherapy that occurs only quite late in this process. I am increasingly convinced that the working through of such childhood trauma in a meaningful way can occur only as part of the working through of negative transference or as a consequence of already having made significant progress in negative transference work. The reason for this is that the borderline patient will otherwise become disorganized or dissociated or will act out on the angry feelings accompanying the recall of such experiences. The patient must first learn to accept and integrate his or her own angry motivations sufficiently that he or she can contain and own angry feelings toward significant others without having self-destructive or pain-numbing responses.

SUMMARY

This chapter extends and modifies observations about the clinical significance of the trauma history of borderline patients. Its overall thesis is that for borderline patients with severe childhood trauma histories, treatment planning should be organized around having a primary clinician whose early role is to help the patient manage his or her everyday life and to diminish its stresses. Frequently, cognitive-behavioral forms of intervention provide the most rapid and safest way to accomplish these goals. Only when such patients' lives have become more stabilized and an alliance with the clinician-manager has been established can exploratory therapy take place. Moreover, the central role that exploratory psychodynamic therapy can have with such patients is the exploration of needed negative transference work in such a way that the borderline patients can own their angry and sadistic motives toward those they depend on before meaningful recollection and working through of childhood trauma can occur.

REFERENCES

Beck AT, Freeman A: Cognitive Therapy of Personality Disorders. New York, Guilford, 1990

Gabbard GO, Horowitz L, Frieswyk SH, et al: The effect of therapist interventions on the therapeutic alliance with borderline patients. J Am Psychoanal Assoc 36:697–727, 1988

Gunderson JG, Chu JA: Treatment implications of past trauma in borderline personality disorder. Harvard Review of Psychiatry 1:75–81, 1993

Gunderson JG, Links PS: Treatment of borderline personality disorder, in Treatment of Psychiatric Disorders: The DSM-IV Edition. Edited by Gabbard GO. Washington, DC, American Psychiatric Press, 1995, pp 2291–2309

Gunderson JG, Sabo AN: The phenomenological and conceptual interface of borderline personality disorder and posttraumatic stress disorder. Am J Psychiatry 150:19–27, 1993

Gunderson JG, Frank AF, Ronningstam EF, et al: Early discontinuance of borderline patients from psychotherapy. J Nerv Ment Dis 177:38–42, 1989

Gunderson JG, Waldinger R, Sabo AN, et al: Stages of change in dynamic psychotherapy with borderline patients: clinical and research implications. Journal of Psychotherapy Practice and Research 2:64–72, 1993

Herman JL, Perry JC, van der Kolk BA: Childhood trauma in borderline personality disorder. Am J Psychiatry 146:490–495, 1989

Howard KI, Kopta SM, Krause MS, et al: The dose-effect relationship in psychotherapy. Am Psychol 41:159–164, 1986

Linehan MM: Dialectical behavior therapy for borderline personality disorder. Bull Menninger Clin 51:261–276, 1987

Linehan MM, Armstrong HE, Suarez A, et al: Cognitive-behavioral treatment of chronically parasuicidal borderline patients. Arch Gen Psychiatry 48:1060–1064, 1991

Links PS, Steiner M, Offord DR, et al: Characteristics of borderline personality disorder: a Canadian study. Can J Psychiatry 33:336–340, 1988

Meichenbaum D: Cognitive Behavior Modification: An Iterative Approach. New York, Plenum, 1977

Skodol AE, Buckley P, Charles E: Is there a characteristic pattern to the treatment history of clinical outpatients with borderline personality? J Nerv Ment Dis 171:405–410, 1983

Waldinger R, Gunderson JG: Effective Psychotherapy With Borderline Patients. New York, Macmillan, 1987

Westen D: Cognitive-behavioral interventions in the psychoanalytic psychotherapy of borderline personality disorders. Clinical Psychology Review 11:211–230, 1991

Young JE: Cognitive Therapy for Personality Disorders: A Schema-Focused Approach. Sarasota, FL, Professional Resource Press, 1990

Zanarini MC, Gunderson JG, Marino MF, et al: Childhood experiences of borderline patients. Compr Psychiatry 30:18–25, 1989

Index

*Page numbers printed in **boldface** type refer to tables.*

Adjective Checklist (ACL), 151
Adolescent Attachment Interview, 73
Adult Attachment Interview, 73
Affective dysregulation, 119, 121–122
Affective lability, 1
Aggression, 2–3
Ambivalent attachment
adult volunteer sample study, 79–86
borderline phenomena and, 74
female undergraduate sample study, 74–79, 83–86
defined, 74, 75, **75**
vulnerability to BPD, 75–78
Amnesia, for trauma, 133
Analysis of variance (ANOVA), 96, 97, 187
Antisocial personality disorder (ASPD)
compared to BPD, 2, 8, 31
increasing odds of developing BPD, 58, 61–62

in prison population, 49, 54
Attachment figure, 73
Attachment theory
classifications and diagnosis, **75, 76, 81**
described, 72–74, 88–89
Attention deficit/ hyperactivity disorder (ADHD), 169, 172, 173, 176
Avoidant attachment, 74, 75, **75,** 79–84
Axis II disorders, other. *See also* Borderline personality disorder (BPD)
BPD and, 1, 2
and neurodevelopmental vulnerability, 11
distinguished from BPD, 31, 32
outpatient control subjects with, 8
parental relationships and, 5

Bed-wetting, 51
Biological risk factors, 25, 205–208
Biosocial theory, 203, 204–214

Biparental neglect, 37–38, 151
Borderline personality
    disorder (BPD). *See also*
    Axis II disorders, other;
    Childhood sexual abuse
    adult diagnostic factors,
        24, 34–35
    anxious attachments, 72,
        88–89
    Axis II disorders
        distinguished from,
        31, 32
    biosocial theory, 203,
        204–214, 220
    characteristics, 42, **58**
    childhood abuse,
        prevalence in, **7**,
        10–11
    childhood experiences
        related to, 45–46
    clinician-manager's role,
        227–228
    CNS dysfunction and,
        174–176
    cognitive-behavioral
        interventions,
        231–233
    current views on, 225–226
    developmental
        impairment and, 172
    diagnosis classification
        schemes, 192
    disordered childhood
        attachment patterns, 11
    dissociation and, 96,
        100–104, 140
    follow-up assessments in
        patients with history
        of CSA, 182–183

heightened risk of, in first-
    degree relatives, 118
major depressive disorder
    and, 136–137
neurological dysfunction
    as a predictor of,
    173–174
neurological variables,
    171, 170
organicity and, 166, 174
pathogenesis
    first-generation studies,
        3–6
    psychodynamic theories,
        2–3
    second-generation
        studies, 6–10
    third-generation studies,
        10–12
pathognomonic
    symptoms, 107
patients not sexually
    abused, 40
personality disorders and, 10
in prison population, 54
psychosocial models, 176
psychotherapy, 157
recovery time, 198–199, 200
research limitations,
    15–17, 41–42
risk factors associated with
    diagnosis, **35**
self-mutilation and, 116
severity of symptoms,
    86–88
sociotherapies, 229–231
studies of pathological
    childhood factors, in
    etiology of

Borderline personality disorder
(BPD) *(continued)*
methodology, 30–32
results, 32–41, **33–35**
role of childhood sexual
abuse in, 29–30
symptoms
DSM-III-R criteria,
192–193
neurological dysfunction
and, 165
sexual abuse and,
138–140
theories, 1–2
therapeutic alliance,
228–229
treatment strategies,
226–227
vulnerable neurological
substrate, 172
Borderline psychopathology,
24, 181
Brain
frontal lobe dysfunction, 176
hemispheric intercom-
munication, 123
injury, 172–173
left anterior dysfunction,
175–176
minimal brain dysfunction
(MBD), 165, 175
neurodevelopmental
deficits and BPD, 173

Carbamazepine treatment, 124
Caretakers. *See* Childhood
sexual abuse
Central nervous system (CNS)
acquired dysfunction, 172

MSAD NHTI assessment
of, 168
neurological predisposition,
174–176
relevance to BPD, 173
vulnerability, 169
Childhood. *See also*
Childhood physical
abuse; Childhood
sexual abuse
defined, 52
disordered childhood
attachment patterns, 11
pathological experiences
neurological
abnormalities and,
176–177
study findings, 31, **33,
34,** 37
questionnaires about
Childhood Antecedents
Questionnaire, 185
Revised Childhood
Experiences
Questionnaire,
31–32
and self-mutilation
childhood factors,
113–115, 118–120,
122
Childhood Antecedents
Questionnaire (CAQ),
185
Childhood physical abuse.
See also Borderline
personality disorder
(BPD); Childhood
sexual abuse
defined, 52

Childhood physical abuse
    (continued)
  intrafamilial, 17
  low rate of physical
      neglect and, 9
  overall rate of, 22
Childhood sexual abuse. See
    also Borderline
    personality disorder
    (BPD); Childhood
    physical abuse
  age of occurrence, 51–52
  by caretakers, 8–10, 16, 20,
      113, 114, **114, 115**
  clinical relevance,
      155–156
  defined, 19
  DES scores related to, 97
  dissociation and self-
      mutilation studies
    compared to other
        studies, 100–104
    methodology, 95
    research, 93–95
    research limitations,
        103–104
    results, 96–100
  early memories and
      malevolent object
      representations, 141
  follow-up studies
    abused group in,
        184–185, 193,
        197–198
    advantages, 183
    data analysis, 187
    diagnostic tools, 184,
        186–187
    implications, 199–200

improvement over time
    among subjects,
    187–192
  limitations, 199
  methodology, 186–187
  nonabused group in,
      185, 196, 198
  real-time prospective
      follow-up study,
      182, 183–186
  results, 192–199
history of abuse, in adult
    volunteer sample, **86**
initial effects, 135
intrafamilial, 151
invalidation, abuse as
    example of, 211–214
long-term aftereffects, 181,
    197, 200
parameters, **21,** 22, 23–26
predictors of long-term
    sequelae, 15–17,
    135–136
prevalence, **7,** 10–11
psychopathology in adults
    and, 24, 181
psychotherapy, 157
rates by perpetrator, **20**
role in BPD, 71–72, 174–176
self-destructiveness and,
    113–115
severity, 145–155
survivors, elevated rates of
    BPD among, 2
women's disorders,
    etiological factor in, 12
Chronic dysfunctional anger, 78
Chronic dysphoria, 1, 140
Clinician-manager, 227–228

Cognitive-behavior therapy,
124–125, 215–216,
231–233
Cognitive deficit, 230
Comorbidity, 55, 177
Criminal offenses, 54

Daughters, turbulent
attachments to
mothers, 76–77
Deliberate injury, 142, 143.
See also Self-mutilation
Depression
compared to BPD, 174
memories and, 133
Derealization, 140
Developmental impairment,
172, 175
Diagnostic Interview for
Borderlines (DIB)
CSA follow-up study, use
in, 184, 186
determining predictors of
items in, **149**
Impulse section, 109
mean scores
items and section scores,
190–191, 194
in University of Michigan
study, 136, 140, 146
Diagnostic Interview for
Personality Disorders
(DIPD), 18–19
Diagnostic Interview
Schedule (DIS), 49–50
Dialectical behavior therapy
(DBT), 215, 216–220
Dichotomous thinking, 230,
232

Disordered childhood
attachment patterns,
11. *See also* Attachment
theory
Dissociation
biosocial theory and, 207
BPD and, 96, 100–104, 140
measures, 95
psychological risk factors,
96–100
PTSD and, 93–94
self-mutilation and, 11
study results, 96–100
trauma spectrum
disorders and, 2
Dissociative Experiences Scale
(DES), 93–94, **95, 96**
Divorce, 3, 4
and mother-daughter
relationships, 85
Dopaminergic systems, 123
DSM-III-R
BPD diagnosis, 80
criteria cluster, 18
mean scores
individual criteria, **189**
Dynamic psychotherapy,
227, 233–235
Dysfunctional anger, 78
Dysphoria, chronic, 1, 140

Early memories, 141–145
Early Memories Test, 141, 143
Electroencephalographic
(EEG) abnormalities,
123, 175, 206
Emotion dysregulation, 205,
207, 208, 216
Emotional development, 206

Environmental events, 207
Epidemiologic Catchment
    Area (ECA), 54

False memory syndrome, 132
Familial Experience
    Interview (FEI), 138
Family environment,
    150–156, 206, 211, 213
Family Environment Scale
    (FES), 152–155
Family violence, 58, 60
Fathers. *See also* Parents
    abuse by, 9, **86**
    sexual, 9, 20–21, **20,** 131,
        152, 208, 215 (case)
    disturbed involvement
        with, 5–6
    relationship with, 5, 6, 151,
        166
    separation from and loss
        of, 4
Female patients
    age at onset of suicidal
        behavior, 114
    CSA study
        methodology, 15–20
        results, 20–26
    dissociation and self-
        mutilation studies
        compared to other
            studies, 100–104
        methodology, 95–100
        research, 93–95
        results, 96–100
    imprisoned for felony, 11,
        47, 48–59
    psychological risk factors
        and DES scores, **97**

Women Inmates' Health
    Study (WIHS)
    answering "yes" on
        dichotomous
        variables, **57**
    diagnosis groups, **56**
    research strengths and
        limitations, 64–65
    results, 53–65
    risk factors for BPD, 47
    study design, 48–53
Frontal lobe dysfunction, 176

Global Assessment Scale
    (GAS), 183

"Hyperactivating"
    interpersonal
    strategies, 78

Impact of Events Scale (IES),
    50, 55
Impulse spectrum disorder, 2
Incest. *See also* Childhood
    sexual abuse
    father-daughter, 16, 23, 131
    and PTSD, 49
    victims, and
        self-destructive
        behavior, 119
Inner object world, 141
Invalidating environment,
    204, 208–214

Learning disabilities, 173
Lifetime Borderline
    Symptom Index (LBSI),
    110
Limbic system dysfunction, 123

Linehan's Dialectical
Behavior Therapy,
11–12, 215–220
Linehan's Suicidal Behaviors
Questionnaire, 187,
193, **195**
Logistic regression
advantages, 52–53
determining CNS
vulnerability, 169
in multivariate analyses
of BPD, 35, 51
of self-mutilation,
dissociation, and
psychological risk
factors, **99**
of self-mutilation and
psychological risk
factors, 98
results, 59–65
testing for possible
confounding data,
143–144
for vulnerable CNS
substrate, 170

Major depressive disorder
(MDD), 136–137
Malevolent object
representations,
141–145
Mayman's Early Memories
Test, 142
McLean Hospital (Belmont,
Massachusetts), study,
31
McLean Study of Adult
Development (MSAD),
168

Medical University of South
Carolina, 50
Minimal brain dysfunction
(MBD), 165, 175
Minnesota Multiphasic
Personality Inventory
(MMPI), 137, 150
Mothers. *See also* Parents
disturbed involvement, 5–6
and divorce, in
mother-daughter
relationships, 85
drug or alcohol use by, 172
intrauterine effects on
emotional
development, 206
maternal inconsistency,
76–78
of preborderline children, 3
MSAD Neurodevelopmental
History and
Temporolimbic
Interview (MSAD
NHTI), 168
Multicolinearity, 35
Multidrug double-blind
crossover study,
123–124
Multiple linear regressions,
153, **154**, 155
Multiple personality
disorder (MPD),
2, 197
Multiple regressions
childhood abuse/neglect
variables and
self-destructive
behavior, **114, 115,
116**

Multiple regressions (continued)
    multiple linear regressions,
        153, **154**, 155
    psychological risk factors
        and, 96, **97**
Multivariate analyses
    of BPD, 57–59
    for CSA, 23
    determining significant
        findings, 10
    nonpredictive variables in
        regression model,
        62–63
    potential predispositional
        factors, 51–53
    predictive variables in
        regression model,
        59–62
    psychological risk factors
        in, 17
    self-mutilation,
        dissociation, and
        psychological risk
        factors, 98–100
    self-mutilation and
        psychological risk
        factors, 98

Neurodevelopmental
    abnormalities, 123
Neurological dysfunction
    limbic system, 207
    neurobehavioral model,
        166
    related to neglectful or
        abusive
        environment, 176
    research, 165–168
    risk factors, 173–174

study
    compared with other
        studies, 173–174
    limitations and
        conclusions, 178
    methodology, 168–169
    questions, 168
    results, 167, 169–173,
        174–177
Neuropsychological testing, 206
Neurosis, 5
New York State Psychiatric
    Institute, 182
Nonpatient samples, 46. See also
    Females, prison inmates
North Carolina, Women
    Inmates' Health Study
    (WIHS). See Women
    Inmates' Health Study
    (WIHS)

Organicity, 166, 174

Paranoid schizophrenia, 5
Parasuicidal behavior, 215
Parental Bonding Index
    (PBI), 19–20, 96, 151
Parents
    Axis II Disorder and, 5
    biparental neglect, 37–38, 151
    chronic dysfunctional
        anger toward, 78
    disturbed parental
        involvement, 4–6
    divorce, 4
    illness, 4
    psychoeducation for,
        229–230
    separation, 3–4, 22, 33

Peabody Picture Vocabulary
 Test (PPVT), 185
Personality Disorders
 Program, Department
 of Psychiatry,
 University of Michigan
 Medical Center, 131
Posttraumatic stress disorder
 (PTSD)
 assessment criteria, 49, 50
 compared to BPD, 2, 24, 30
 dissociative symptoms
  and, 93
 increasing odds of
  developing BPD, 58,
  61, 136
 in prison population, 54–55
 in women prison inmates, 48
Promiscuity, 140
Pseudo-adult behavior, 156
Psychiatric illness, 193–196,
 197–198
Psychological risk factors
 dissociation and, 96–100
 influencing CSA and BPD, 25
 self-mutilation and, 98, **99**
Psychological trauma, 50, 54, 67
Psychopathology, 196, 225
Psychosocial models, of BPD,
 176
Psychotherapy, 39–41, 157
 dynamic, 227, 233–235
 supportive, 231

Rape, 78, 215. *See also*
 Childhood sexual
 abuse; Incest
 and Childhood Antecedents
 Questionnaire, 184

and long-term outcome, of
 subjects, 182
and PTSD, 49
Research Diagnostic Criteria
 (RDC), 137, 184, 186
Retrospective sexual abuse
 data, 132–135
Revised Childhood Experiences
 Questionnaire, 31–32
Revised Diagnostic Interview
 for Borderlines (DIB-R)
 continuous variables, 110
 measuring self-mutilation, 95
 separating borderline
  from nonborderline
  personality
  disorders, 18, 31
Revised Diagnostic Interview
 for Personality Disorders
 (DIPD-R), 31, 49
Rorschach test, 150
Rosenberg Self-Esteem Scale,
 137

Schedule for Affective
 Disorders and
 Schizophrenia (SADS),
 184
Schedule for Affective
 Disorders and
 Schizophrenia—Lifetime
 Interval Version
 (SADS-LI), 186
Schizophrenia, 1, 5, 174
Secure/ambivalent
 attachment, 74, 75
Secure attachment
 borderline phenomena
  and, 74

Secure attachment *(continued)*
    defined, 75
    emotional resilience, 78–79
Secure/avoidant attachment,
    74, 75
Self-destructive behavior. *See*
    Axis II disorders, other;
    Childhood sexual
    abuse; Self-mutilation
Self-esteem, Rosenberg Scale,
    137
Self-mutilation. *See also*
    Suicidal behavior
    affective dysregulation
        leading to, 119
    age at onset, 111, 117–118
    biological aspects, 123–124
    characteristic childhood
        experiences, 122
    childhood factors,
        113–115, 118–120
    DES scores, **99**
    dissociation and, 11
    extremes of, 113
    as form of communication,
        120–121
    lifetime patterns of, 116, 125
    measured on DIB-R, 95
    number of attempts, 114
    psychological risk factors, 98
    research, 107, 110
    super self-mutilators, 113,
        117–118
    symptoms, 94–95
    treatment modes
        with carbamazepine, 124
        cognitive-behavior
            therapy, 124–125
        integrative approach, 125

Self-reflection, 124
Separation-individuation, 3
Sexual abuse. *See also*
    Childhood sexual abuse
    coding severity of, 146
    defined, 138
    rape, 78, 215
    reenactments of, 157
    retrospective data,
        132–135
    vulnerable CNS substrate
        and, 177
Single-parent families, 4
Sociodemographic
    characteristics, 46, 53–54
Socioeconomic status (SES)
    measure, 74
Sociotherapies, 229–231
Splitting, 230, 231
Statistics. *See* Logistic
    regression; Multiple
    regressions; Multivariate
    analyses
Stone, Michael, 131
Structured Clinical Interview
    for DSM-III-R Axis I
    Disorders (SCID-I), 31, 48
Structured Clinical Interview
    for DSM-III-R
    Personality Disorders
    (SCID-II), 80
Structured Interview for
    DSM-III-R Personality
    Disorders (SIDP-R),
    186–187
Suggestibility, 133
Suicidal behavior. *See also*
    Self-mutilation
    age at onset, 107–108, 114, 115

contingency planning for, 124
linked to CSA, 214–216
parasuicidal behavior, 215
prevalence of, 112
super suicide attempters, 113
Suicidal Behaviors
Questionnaire (SBQ),
187, 193, **195**
Super self-mutilators, 113,
117–118. *See also*
Self-mutilation
Super suicide attempters, 113.
See also Self-mutilation;
Suicidal behavior
Supportive psychotherapy, 231

Therapeutic alliance, 228–229
Therapy modes
cognitive-behavior
therapy, 124–125,
215–216, 231–233
dialectical behavior
therapy, 215, 216–220
Linehan's Dialectical
Behavior Therapy,
11–12, 215–220
psychotherapy, 39–41
dynamic, 227, 233–235
supportive, 231
sociotherapies, 229–231
therapeutic alliance,
228–229
Transactional theory, 213–214
Trauma-induced
neurodevelopmental
abnormalities, 123
Trauma spectrum disorder, 2
Traumatic memories, 133

Univariate analyses, 98
University of Michigan
Medical Center,
Personality Disorders
Program, 131
University of Michigan studies
BPD symptoms and sexual
abuse, 138–140
early memories, sexual
abuse, and
malevolent object
representations,
141–145
methodology, 136–138
severity of sexual abuse
and BPD symptoms,
145–150
and family environment,
150–155

Validating environment, 209
Vulnerable CNS substrate,
169, 170, 171, 177
Vulnerable neurological
substrate, 172

Women. *See* Daughters;
Female patients;
Mothers
Women Inmates' Health
Study (WIHS)
answering "yes" on
dichotomous
variables, **57**
diagnosis groups, **56**
research limitations, 64–65
results, 53–65
risk factors for BPD, 47
study design, 48–53